PRACTICAL KINESIOLOGY
FOR THE
PHYSICAL THERAPIST
ASSISTANT

PRACTICAL KINESIOLOGY FOR THE PHYSICAL THERAPIST ASSISTANT

Edited by Jeff G. Konin, MEd, ATC, MPT

Illustrations by Ira A. Grunther, CMI

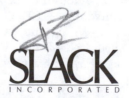

SLACK
INCORPORATED

6900 Grove Road • Thorofare, NJ 08086

Publisher: John H. Bond
Editorial Director: Amy E. Drummond
Associate Editor: Jennifer L. Stewart

Konin, Jeff G.
 Practical kinesiology for the physical therapist assistant/edited by Jeff G. Konin.
  p. cm.
 Includes bibliographical references and index.
 ISBN 1-55642-299-7 (alk. paper)
 1. Kinesiology. 2. Physical therapist assistants. I. Konin, Jeff G.
 [DNLM: 1. Allied Health Personnel. 2. Kinesiology, Applied.
 3. Physical Therapy--methods. WE 103 P8955 1999]
 QP301.P73 1999
 612.7'6--dc21
 DNLM/DLC
 for Library of Congress   NWSt

            IAHQ 3409   99-20311
                          CIP

Printed in the United States of America
Published by: SLACK Incorporated
   6900 Grove Road
   Thorofare, NJ 08086-9447 USA
   Telephone: 609-848-1000 or 856-848-1000
   Fax: 609-853-5991 or 856-853-5991
   http://www.slackinc.com

The work SLACK Incorporated publishes is peer reviewed. Prior to publication, recognized leaders in the field, educators, and clinicians provide important feedback on the concepts and content that we publish. We welcome feedback on this work.

Contact SLACK Incorporated for more information about other books in this field or about the availability of our books from distributors outside the United States.

Last digit is print number: 10 9 8 7 6 5 4 3 2 1

DEDICATION

To my mother, Lenore, and my son, Kyle James,
who have enabled me to comprehend the true meaning of life.

CONTENTS

ACKNOWLEDGMENTS

During the course of any project that takes nearly 4 years to complete, one develops a special appreciation for the final outcome. This outcome not only brings with it a sense of accomplishment, but also a dimension of relief and fulfillment in knowing that the fruits of the labor will lead to the nourishing of tomorrow's professionals.

Most of the credit for developing this textbook from a simple idea belongs to Amy Drummond, Editorial Director at SLACK Incorporated. From its inception, Amy has played a vital role in recognizing the importance of such a text. In doing so, her valuable guidance throughout this process was the driving force behind our goal of teaching kinesiology to physical therapist assistant students in a practical and understandable way. Having the opportunity to work with such an extremely professional and wonderful person as Amy Drummond is something no author should miss out on.

Many other individuals from SLACK Incorporated must also be mentioned for the roles that they have played. John Bond, in his role as Publisher, has such a special way of communicating throughout the many trials and tribulations of academic textbook writing that an author can always be assured that he is ultimately concerned with publishing nothing less than the best possible product. A good portion of publishing happens behind the scenes where valuable players are often overlooked. I am indebted to such individuals as Jennifer Stewart for her editorial direction and support, to Jenifer Neiswender and Mary Ellen O'Connor for their efforts in marketing this textbook, and especially to Debra Christy, whose editorial role oftentimes turned her into a "jack of all trades." As always, the receptiveness and support of Peter Slack and the confidence that he has given to his staff must be commended.

The main reason for putting these ideas into textbook form came as a result of frustration in teaching kinesiology to physical therapist assistant students without a good tool that showed the relationship between movement and physical therapy. A good portion of the concepts have been delivered in a format that has been compiled from ideas and suggestions of previous students. In addition, the contributions of others have been greatly appreciated. Thanks to Julie Moyer Knowles, who not only contributed to the text by writing Chapter 7, but who also shared in the enthusiasm of developing a book for the sole purpose of making learning more understandable. Also, thanks to Gina Konin, Kirk Peck, Gary Shankman, and Dennis Whitesel, all of whom added valuable criticism to the early drafts of the text. A special thanks to Todd Brock, who graciously volunteered to model for most of the photographs, and to Ira Grunther, whose marvelous illustrations have helped to visually demonstrate much of what is truly a three-dimensional topic.

Lastly, a very special "thanks" to my wife Gina, who knows better than anyone else how important this project was to me. Her support, guidance, patience, and love have been the keys to allowing me to complete this long journey while simultaneously fulfilling my role as husband and daddy.

—*Jeff G. Konin, MEd, ATC, MPT*

ABOUT THE EDITOR

Jeff G. Konin, MEd, ATC, MPT is a licensed physical therapist and a certified athletic trainer who currently serves as an instructor in the physical therapist assistant program at the Owens Campus of Delaware Technical and Community College in Georgetown, Del, and President of Coastal Health Consultants, PA in Lewes, Del. Mr. Konin received his Bachelor of Science from Eastern Connecticut State University, a Master of Education from the University of Virginia, and a Master of Physical Therapy from the University of Delaware.

Mr. Konin is also the textbook editor of *Clinical Athletic Training*, and co-editor of *Special Tests For Orthopedic Examination*. He has contributed to numerous textbook chapters, sits on the advisory and/or editorial boards for a number of sports medicine related publications, and has given hundreds of presentations all over the world on various topics related to physical therapy and athletic training. In 1996, he served on the track and field medical staff for the Olympic Games in Atlanta, Ga.

CONTRIBUTING AUTHORS

Scott Biely, MS, PT
Chester County Orthopaedic and Sports Physical Therapy
West Chester, Pennsylvania

Glenn P. Brown, MMSc, PT, ATC, SCS
Smith and Brown, PT
Dover, Delaware

Gina L. Konin, PT, ATC
Vice President, Coastal Health Consultants, PA
Lewes, Delaware

Jeff G. Konin, MEd, ATC, MPT
President, Coastal Health Consultants, PA
Lewes, Delaware

Delaware Technical and Community College
Physical Therapist Assistant Program
Georgetown, Delaware

Julie A. Moyer Knowles, EdD, ATC, PT
Healthsouth at Pike Creek Sports Medicine Center
Wilmington, Delaware

Mary Mundrane-Zweiacher, PT, ATC
Smith and Brown, PT
Dover, Delaware

Kirk M. Peck, MS, PT
Clarkson College Physical Therapist Assistant Program
Omaha, Nebraska

FOREWORD

The study of kinesiology is the cornerstone of the foundational knowledge used by the physical therapist assistant to comprehend the complexity of human motion and to understand the principles upon which treatment decisions for individuals with musculoskeletal disorders are based. *Practical Kinesiology for the Physical Therapist Assistant* is a comprehensive text written specifically for the physical therapist assistant to provide such foundational knowledge. This text contains the requisite components for the study of kinesiology, with nicely organized chapters detailing terminology, biomechanical principles, joint structure and function, and muscle structure and function. In six chapters covering the joints of the extremities, the requisite components are applied in the descriptions of the structure and function of individual joints. These components are further integrated in chapters on spine and posture, and gait. A chapter on principles of tissue repair, not ordinarily contained in a kinesiology textbook, provides a basis for the understanding of the many relevant clinical applications included in each chapter. The inclusion of an appendix containing muscle attachments, actions, and innervations serves as a convenient reference for the student of kinesiology.

The extensive clinical applications provided in each chapter are among the most useful aspects of this text. The clinical applications elucidate relatively complex kinesiological principles and serve to forge a transition between the basic and the clinical sciences. An extensive list of references and suggested readings at the end of each chapter add to the richness of the content and provide validation for the clinical applications.

The comprehensiveness of *Practical Kinesiology for the Physical Therapist Assistant* makes this text applicable to many courses within a curriculum for the preparation of physical therapist assistants. Practicing physical therapist assistant clinicians should also find this text a valuable resource in the clinical setting.

—Elisa M. Zuber, MS, PT
Department of Accreditation
American Physical Therapy Association

PREFACE

Practical Kinesiology for the Physical Therapist Assistant is a collection of didactic and practical sciences specifically designed to meet the educational needs of the physical therapist assistant (PTA) student who is studying movement of the human body. The intent of this educational textbook is to serve as an introduction to kinesiology.

I firmly believe that every student should incorporate a well-rounded scientific foundation of biomechanics prior to the development of any clinical application of physical therapy skills. It is only then that one can begin to understand, and more importantly appreciate, the role of the therapeutic intervention.

In preparing this text, I have carefully tended to the current needs of the PTA, whose responsibilities as a member of the rehabilitation team have grown considerably over the years. Inclusion of the topics covered in this text reflect a solid basis from which a student can establish a comfortable body of knowledge in the area of human movement.

Historically, physical therapist assistant educators have been exposed to a library of textbooks in this subject area, only to be less than satisfied with the ability to match the textbook's presentation style with the instructor's curricular needs and level of delivery. In the past, we have taught kinesiology to PTA students through the use of books specifically designed for physical therapists. The act of "altering" these texts for PTA education is not only difficult, it is also wrong. Other texts I have come across have identified the intent to deliver material of this matter to PTA students, yet in my opinion have come up short in reaching that goal.

Practical Kinesiology is not designed to be an all-inclusive anatomical text, nor has it been written to deliver information that has no relevance to the practice of physical therapy by physical therapist assistants. Rather, the goal of *Practical Kinesiology* is to provide the PTA student with a body of knowledge sufficient enough to recognize how normal human movement occurs and how interruptions to normalcy can lead to pathological conditions.

Each chapter follows a consistent format to allow for reader simplicity. All chapters begin with a set of learning objectives that identify the major points of emphasis for the subject matter. These objectives are presented in both didactic and practical formats so that each student can not only recognize the importance of learning the material according to the textbook-related facts, but also as this information relates to practical implementation.

Chapters addressing individual and specific anatomical locations of the body provide an overview of relevant osteology, musculature, joint structure, neural innervation and vascular supply. In addition, attention is placed on the arthrokinetics and arthrokinematics of the related areas. Common pathology of these areas is also described with respect to mechanism of injury as well as some general rehabilitation guidelines.

At the conclusion of each chapter the reader will find a set of study questions that combine the didactic and practical learning areas. Questions have been specifically designed to challenge the reader to identify pertinent responses that can be directly transferred into clinical practice.

Chapter 1 outlines and explains the various terminology associated with human movement. This is the very hallmark by which the entire text follows. A clear understanding of the language is essential to any discussion involving physical therapy. I have attempted to point out the fact that many definitions of human movement are interchangeable and often referred to differently by various clinicians, thus emphasizing the importance of some sense of familiarity on behalf of the reader to recognize relevant terms.

Chapter 2 discusses the factors related to biomechanics, such as forces, lever arms, and resistance. Here, the reader is introduced not only to how forces such as muscles, gravity, and friction relate to movement, but more importantly, how these forces affect therapeutic intervention. Practical objectives and study questions challenge the reader to think from a clinical perspective.

Chapter 3 addresses joint structure and function of the human body. Emphasis is placed on both mobility and immobility, and the various ways in which joints respond to the stresses placed against them. Concepts of rehabilitation are discussed with respect to joint function.

Chapter 4 takes a unique look at muscle structure and function. Terms such as tenodesis, passive insufficiency, and active insufficiency are explained in great detail. The different types of muscle classification and muscle contraction are demonstrated for the reader in illustrations and photographs. Clinical relevance and contraindications of various muscular contractions are discussed and related to daily considerations.

Perhaps of all the chapters in this text, Chapter 5 stands out as one that is unprecedented, yet quite needed in the educational curriculum of the physical therapist assistant. This chapter discusses the principles of tissue repair. The phases of healing, recognition of cardinal signs of inflammation, and the healing properties of specific tissue (including bone, ligament, cartilage, muscle, and nerve) are discussed as they relate to rehabilitation.

Chapters 6 through 12 take a focused look at the shoulder, elbow, wrist and hand, spine, hip, knee, and ankle and foot regions of the body. Each chapter is filled with illustrations and photographs that attempt to provide the reader with a graphic version of the key points of emphasis.

Chapter 13 takes a look at human gait. Perhaps this is the one area of the text that has provided the greatest challenge. It is not accepted in any body of writing within the profession of physical therapy that physical therapist assistants perform gait analysis or evaluation of gait deviations. Thus, one might question the inclusion of this content. It is my belief that the PTA should be familiar with what is considered to be normal gait and the terminology with which it is associated. Furthermore, a PTA is expected to report any changes in a patient's performance, especially those that are adverse in nature, to the supervising physical therapist. Therefore, it becomes imperative that a practicing PTA become familiar with recognizable changes in one's gait. The attempt to include this chapter is not to identify the process of evaluation, but instead to allow for visualization of abnormal pathology.

I do encourage the reader to use this text with an accompanying complete anatomical reference. However, an appendix of muscles is included, each inclusive of the muscle's proximal attachment, distal attachment, primary action, and nerve innervation. A second appendix is also provided as a reference for solving biomechanical equations of the trigonometry type.

This text has been designed by physical therapists who have both clinical experience and academic teaching experience in accredited physical therapist assistant curriculums. Thus, the content matter, the writing style, and the purposeful inclusion of practical considerations directly relate to the needs of the PTA students as seen by the author and contributors based on our experiences.

The science of kinesiology is fairly straightforward. How well a student learns the principles of human movement depends partly on the delivery of the material by a knowledgeable and enthusiastic instructor. No textbook can take the place of a successful teacher. As one who passionately enjoys teaching kinesiology, I can attest to the fact that each instructor has worked diligently to develop his or her own style of teaching methods. Thus, this textbook, or any other for that matter, may not match to perfection the goals of an instructor. However, I believe that it can serve as a very valuable foundation that will allow students the opportunity to learn in a practical manner. Instructors who choose to use this textbook in their curricula are encouraged to use supplemental material and their own idiosyncrasies to further enhance the learning process.

I hope that you will find *Practical Kinesiology for the Physical Therapist Assistant* useful in your delivery of such important and clinically relevant educational information.

—*Jeff G. Konin, MEd, ATC, MPT*

CHAPTER 1

TERMINOLOGY

Jeff G. Konin, MEd, ATC, MPT

OBJECTIVES

After completion of this chapter, the reader will be able to:

DIDACTIC

1. Define kinesiology and biomechanics.
2. Identify common anatomical regions of the body.
3. Recognize the common planes and axes of the body and give examples of each.
4. Describe the various types of movements that occur about the different joints and give an example of each.

PRACTICAL

1. Palpate different anatomical regions of the body.
2. Perform movements in the sagittal, frontal, and coronal planes.

INTRODUCTION

The study of the principles of mechanics and anatomy in relation to human movement is referred to as *kinesiology*. The word is of Greek origin and comprised of two verbs: *kinein*, meaning "to move," and *logos*, meaning "to discourse." When one considers the field of kinesiology, the utilization of disciplines including anatomy, physiology, physics, chemistry, and many other physical sciences cannot be ignored. The ability to bring together the various components from each of these disciplines will determine one's level of understanding kinesiology.

The term *biomechanics* is often described as the study of kinesiology as it affects human movement. Therefore, this text will devote careful attention to biomechanics. More importantly, practical biomechanics, or the ability to understand human movement as it relates to everyday functional activity, will be emphasized. We will attempt to explain the principles of movement and how they relate to assorted structures of the body, as well as their direct effect on the joints at hand.

Grasping the concepts associated with human movement can be a difficult and challenging process. However, with keen insight and focus on basic principles that form the foundation of human movement, the efforts can be quite rewarding. The first step is to become familiar with common terminology associated with kinesiology.

ANATOMICAL REGIONS

Terminology used to describe various regions of the human body can often be ambiguous. For example, it is not uncommon to see the word "head" referred to as the *capitis*. Likewise, the "neck" is the *cervix*, the "trunk" is the *thorax*, and the "limbs" are called *appendages* or *appendiculars*, as well as *extremities*. Since it is an unrealistic task to expect uniformity amongst anatomists and practicing clinicians who have been taught through many different schools, it becomes incumbent upon the reader to become familiar with the different terms used to describe anatomical regions and movements used in this text as well as others.

To begin with, let's discuss what is known as the *anatomical position*. The anatomical position is one in which all directional movements are referred to as in a static position. It consists of an erect posture with eyes looking straight ahead, heels nearly together, and feet pointing slightly

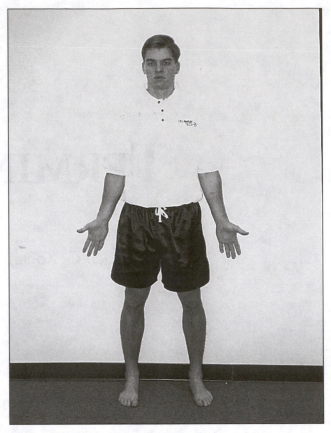

Figure 1-1. Anatomical position.

outward. One's arms are placed at their respective sides with the palms or volar surfaces facing forward or anteriorly (Figure 1-1).

From the anatomical position, the following directional terms are used to describe locations of structures relative to the body (Figures 1-2 and 1-3):

- Anterior: relative to the front surface
- Posterior: relative to the back surface
- Superior: nearer to the head
- Inferior: nearer to the feet
- Medial: nearer to the midline
- Lateral: further away from the midline

With respect to the trunk, the following terms can be used (see Figures 1-2 and 1-3):

- Ventral: relative to the abdominal surface
- Dorsal: relative to the back surface
- Cranial/cephalic: nearer to the head
- Caudal: nearer to the tail end
- Medial: closer to the midline
- Lateral: further away from the midline
- Flexion: forward movement in the sagittal plane
- Extension: backward movement in the sagittal plane

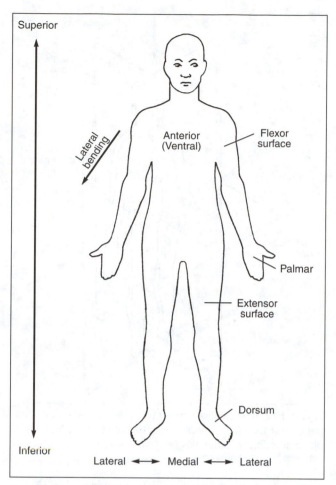

Figure 1-2. Common directional terms used to describe locations of structures relative to the body (anterior view).

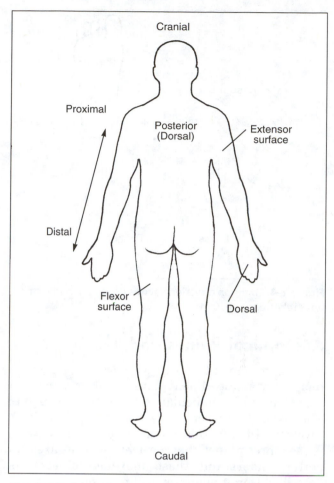

Figure 1-3. Common directional terms used to describe locations of structures relative to the trunk (posterior view).

- Lateral flexion (side bending): movement in the frontal plane to the left or right

With respect to the limbs, the following terms can be used (Figure 1-4):
- Proximal: closer to the trunk
- Distal: further away from the trunk
- Flexor surface: the anterior surface of the upper extremity and the posterior surface of the lower extremity
- Extensor surface: the posterior surface of the upper extremity and the anterior surface of the lower extremity

With respect to the hands and feet, the following terms can be used (see Figure 1-4):
- Palmar/volar surface: the palm surface of the hand
- Dorsum: the posterior surface of the hand and the superior surface of the foot

- Plantar surface: the inferior surface of the foot

Furthermore, the following terms can be used to describe anatomical positions:
- Interior: a structure inside or internal
- Exterior: a structure outside or external
- Ipsilateral: a structure relative to another located on the same side of the body
- Contralateral: a structure relative to another located on the opposite side of the body

All of the previously identified terms are used to describe relatively static positions and should be used when locating a body part in comparison to another part or location. For example, the wrist is not distal. Rather, it is distal when compared to the elbow, with respect to the trunk. Similarly, the knee is not considered to be caudal until compared to a structure such as the hip, which is more proximal to the trunk.

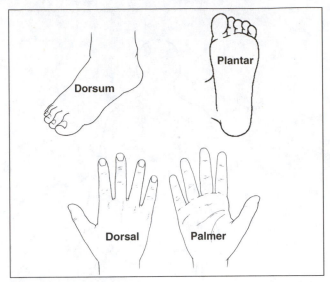

Figure 1-4. Common directional terms used to describe structures relative to the limbs.

Anatomical Planes and Axes

The movement of any joint occurs within an imaginary plane. Each plane revolves about an axis that is perpendicular to the respective plane. The axis is the central point at which a joint revolves. In general, human movement encompasses three planes that move about three axes. To better understand these movements, each is described from the anatomical position.

A *sagittal plane* divides the body into left and right sections. Movement occurring in this plane essentially occurs in the anterior/posterior direction. Movement of this type revolves around a *horizontal* or *transverse axis* (Figure 1-5). Examples of joint movement occurring in the sagittal plane are elbow and knee flexion and extension.

A *frontal* or *coronal plane* is one which divides the body into front and back or anterior and posterior sections. Side-to-side movement, such as side bending of the neck or trunk, occurs in this plane. These types of movements revolve about a *sagittal axis*, or what is more commonly termed an *anterior/posterior axis* (see Figure 1-5).

The third plane existing in human movement is the *horizontal* or *transverse plane*. This plane essentially divides the body into a top and bottom section. Movement in this plane occurs around a *longitudinal axis*, which can be seen as a *vertical axis*. Rotational movements such as internal and external rotation of the glenohumeral joint of the shoulder occur within this plane (see Figure 1-5). Analogous to this type of movement is a ballerina

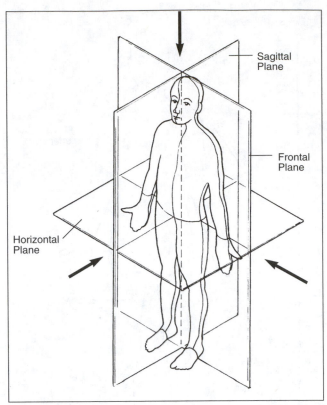

Figure 1-5. Movement occurring through a plane and it's perpendicular axis: (a.) sagittal plane, transverse axis; (b.) frontal plane, anterior/posterior axis; (c.) transverse plane, longitudinal axis.

on her toes spinning around, whereby the movement is occurring in a horizontal plane about a vertical axis.

TERMINOLOGY RELATED TO MOVEMENT OF JOINTS

To clarify and objectively identify movements of the joints, specific terms are used to define each movement that takes place about a joint. Many of the terms are synonymous with multiple joints. However, some terms are used solely to describe the movement of a particular joint. Typically, each described movement also has an antagonistic movement. As described later, these movements may occur actively via a muscular contraction, or they may be passive in nature, whereby an external force produces the movement. This external force may include a machine of some type or may simply be the result of a clinician mobilizing a subject's joint.

The term *flexion* is used to describe a movement that creates a decrease about the joint angle

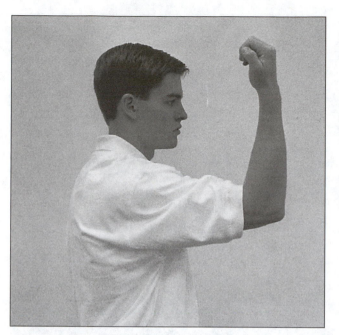

Figure 1-6a. Flexion of the elbow joint.

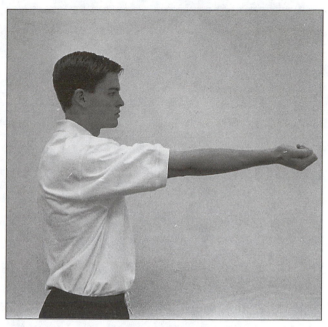

Figure 1-6b. Extension of the elbow joint.

and occurs in the sagittal plane. This can be seen in the elbow for example, in which elbow flexion decreases the angle about the joint (Figure 1-6a). It can also be seen in joints such as the wrist, trunk, hip, knee, and ankle. *Extension*, increasing the joint angle, is the antagonistic movement to flexion of a joint (Figure 1-6b). There is an exception to this definition with respect to angular changes and that is when one looks at the glenohumeral joint. When one measures glenohumeral flexion from the anatomical position, the joint angle actually increases and the angle decreases during extension. When a joint is moved beyond its normal anatomical limitations with respect to flexion and extension, the terms *hyperflexion* and *hyperextension* are used, respectively.

A flexion movement can also occur in a lateral direction, or what is known as *side bending*. This is seen with both the neck and the trunk. With *lateral flexion*, or side bending, the terms "left" or "right" are used to describe the direction of the movement and any measurements that begin with "0" at the anatomical position and increase with bending (Figures 1-7a and 1-7b).

At the ankle, movement in both directions of the sagittal plane are referred to as flexion. Isolated movement toward the dorsum is known as *dorsiflexion*, while movement toward the plantar surface of the foot is called *plantarflexion*. Both occur in the sagittal plane (Figures 1-8a and 1-8b).

Rotation is examined in a similar fashion to side bending, whereas the terms "left" and "right" are used when referring to the neck and trunk. Additionally, when referencing rotation with respect the limbs, the terms *internal* (medial) and *external* (lateral) *rotation* are used. Internal alludes to a movement toward the midline and external away from the midline (Figures 1-9a and 1-9b). Rotation that occurs about a 360º circumference is called *circumduction*. This is typically seen in ball-and-socket joints such as the hip and shoulder (Figure 1-10).

While internal and external rotation can be seen at the forearm, here it is more commonly described as *pronation* and *supination*, respectively. With pronation, the palm is seen moving from a position where it faces upward to where it faces in a downward direction as the radius crosses over the ulna (Figure 1-11a). With supination, the palm is moved into the anatomical position where it faces upward (Figure 1-11b). Pronation and supination are terms that are also used to describe positions of the foot. However, as will be discussed later in the text, this really describes a combination of three different component movements.

Abduction refers to a joint movement in a direction away from the midline of the body (Figure 1-12a). The opposite movement to this is *adduction*, whereby a movement occurs in a direction toward the midline of the body (Figure 1-12b). Abduction and adduction will occur in the frontal plane. Abduction and adduction movements in the

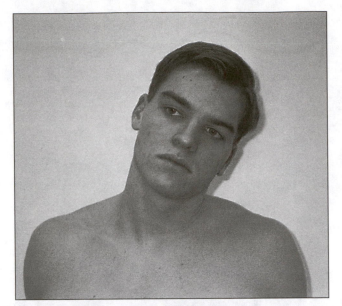

Figure 1-7a. Lateral flexion of the neck.

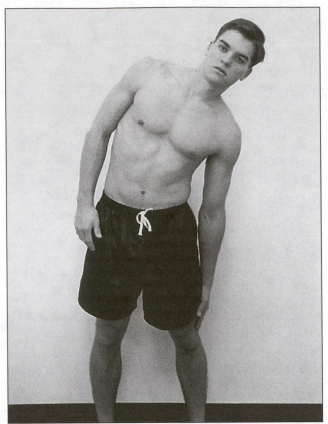

Figure 1-7b. Lateral flexion of the trunk.

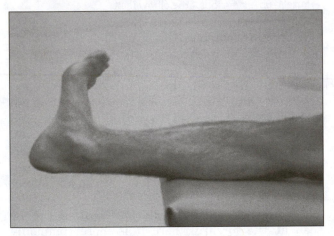

Figure 1-8a. Movement of the ankle: dorsiflexion.

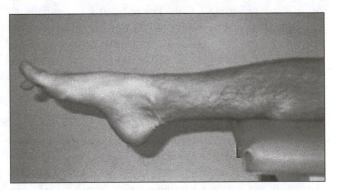

Figure 1-8b. Movement of the ankle: plantarflexion.

horizontal plane are referred to as *horizontal abduction* and *adduction*, as is seen with the glenohumeral joint (Figures 1-13a and 1-13b).

Abduction and adduction that take place at the wrist are more commonly termed *radial* and *ulnar deviation*, respectively. Viewing from the anatomical position, abduction of the wrist involves a movement away from the body in the frontal plane toward the radius (Figure 1-14a). Adduction involves a movement toward the body in a direction toward the ulna (Figure 1-14b).

Protraction and *retraction* are directional terms used to describe movements in the forward and backward directions. These terms are used specifically to describe movement of the scapula as it relates to the thorax (Figure 1-15). When one reaches forward, the scapula protracts. Retraction of the scapula is seen when one pinches the shoulder blades together, or it can be identified pathologically when there is an insult to the neuromuscular structures assisting with the movement of the scapulothoracic joint, as will be discussed in Chapter 6.

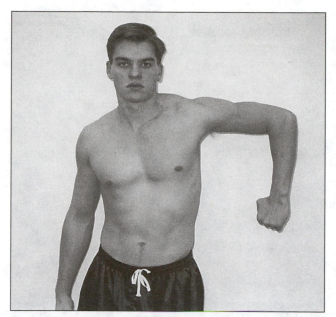

Figure 1-9a. Rotation movement at the limbs: internal rotation.

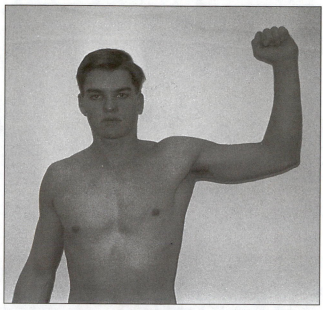

Figure 1-9b. Rotation movement at the limbs: external rotation.

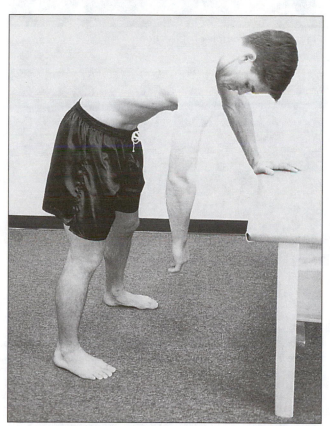

Figure 1-10. Circumduction as seen at the glenohumeral joint of the shoulder.

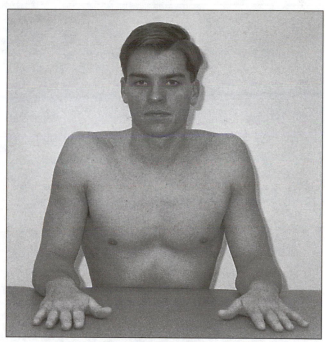

Figure 1-11a. Pronation of the forearm.

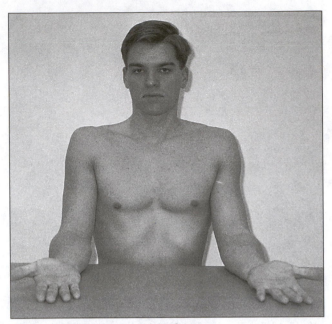

Figure 1-11b. Supination of the forearm.

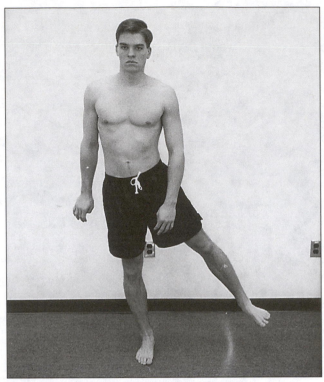

Figure 1-12a. Example of abduction.

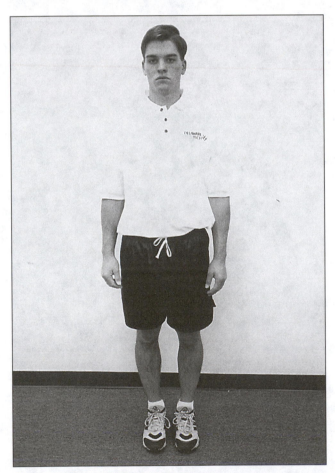

Figure 1-12b. Example of adduction.

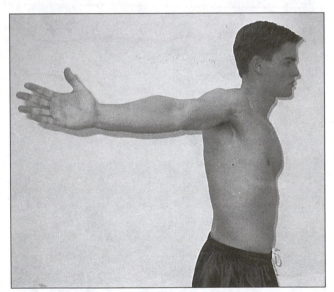

Figure 1-13a. Example of horizontal abduction.

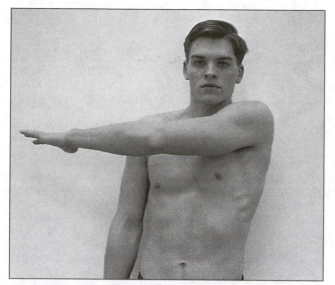

Figure 1-13b. Example of horizontal adduction.

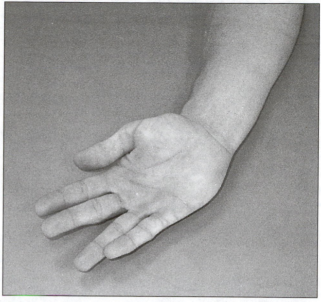

Figure 1-14a. At the wrist, radial deviation (abduction) is viewed from the anatomical position and occurs in a frontal plane.

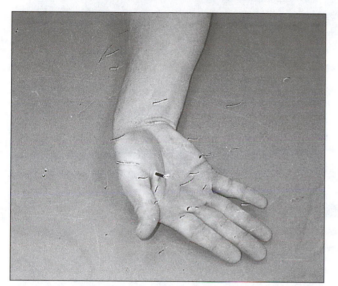

Figure 1-14b. At the wrist, ulnar deviation (adduction) is viewed from the anatomical position and occurs in a frontal plane.

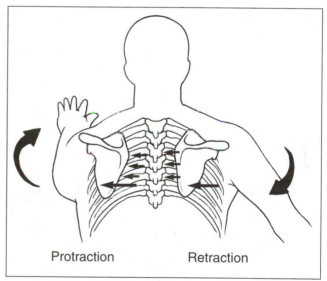

Protraction   Retraction

Figure 1-15. Protraction and retraction as seen in the scapula.

PALPATION OF ANATOMICAL SURFACES

When studying anatomical terminology and the movements associated with the structures, it is helpful to palpate muscles, tendons, and joints in an attempt to better appreciate what is actually occurring. To do so, the examiner might incorporate a list of the following palpation principles:

1. Have the subject in a comfortable and relaxed position.
2. Support the body part being examined.
3. Be sure any surrounding musculature is in a relaxed position.
4. Expose the area for optimal observation.
5. Use the pads of the index and middle fingers to palpate (Figure 1-16).
6. Use a sensitive but firm touch.

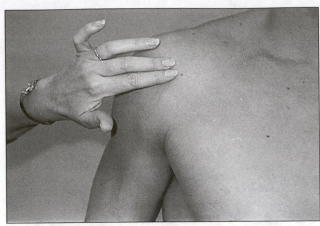

Figure 1-16. Palpation using the pads of the fingers.

Suggested Reading

Daniels L, Worthingham C. *Muscle Testing Techniques of Manual Examination.* 5th ed. Philadelphia, Pa: WB Saunders; 1986.

Kisner C, Colby LA. *Therapeutic Exercise: Foundations and Techniques.* 3rd ed. Philadelphia, Pa: FA Davis Company; 1996.

Lippert L. *Clinical Kinesiology for Physical Therapist Assistants.* 2nd ed. Philadelphia, Pa: FA Davis Company; 1994.

Magee DJ. *Orthopedic Physical Assessment.* 2nd ed. Philadelphia, Pa: WB Saunders; 1992.

Moore K. *Clinically Oriented Anatomy.* 2nd ed. Baltimore, Md: Williams & Wilkins; 1985.

Norkin C, Levangie P. *Joint Structure and Function: A Comprehensive Analysis.* Philadelphia, Pa: FA Davis Company; 1983.

Norkin C, White D. *Measurement of Joint Motion: A Guide of Goniometry.* Philadelphia, Pa: FA Davis Company; 1985.

Pratt NE. *Clinical Musculoskeletal Anatomy.* Philadelphia, Pa: JB Lippincott; 1991.

Rasch PJ. *Kinesiology and Applied Anatomy.* 7th ed. Philadelphia, Pa: Lea & Febiger; 1989.

Wadsworth CT. *Manual Examination and Treatment of the Spine and Extremities.* Baltimore, Md: Williams & Wilkins; 1988.

1. Define kinesiology. How many different disciplines can you think of that would contribute to kinesiology?

2. List another anatomical term that can be used to describe each of the following regions:
   a. Head
   b. Neck
   c. Trunk
   d. Limb

3. Demonstrate the anatomical position.

4. Using the correct anatomical terminology, fill in the blank with the appropriate term:
   a. The hand is _____ to the elbow.
   b. The right knee is _____ to the right shoulder.
   c. The eyes are _____ to the mouth.
   d. The bicep muscle is on the _____ surface.
   e. The quadricep muscle group is on the _____ surface.
   f. The sole of the foot is referred to as the _____ surface.
   g. The ulna is _____ to the radius.
   h. The pectoralis muscle is on the _____ side of the trunk.

5. Demonstrate a joint movement that takes place in each of the following planes:
   a. Sagittal
   b. Frontal
   c. Transverse
   Each of these movements is perpendicular to what axis?

6. List the plane and axis in which each of the following joint movements occur:
   a. Elbow flexion and extension
   b. Hip abduction and adduction
   c. Pronation and supination of the forearm
   d. Trunk side bending
   e. Cervical rotation
   f. Glenohumeral internal and external rotation
   g. Radial and ulnar deviation

7. Name a joint that may be prone to hyperextension or hyperflexion. Can you explain why this may occur?

8. List five principles recommended when palpating anatomical surfaces.

9. Practice palpating the following structures during joint movements:
   a. Patella
   b. Medial malleolus of the tibia
   c. Greater trochanter of the femur
   d. Lateral epicondyle of the humerus
   e. Muscles of the neck during rotation and side bending
   f. Tendons of the wrist
   g. Bicep muscle during elbow flexion

CHAPTER 2

BIOMECHANICAL PRINCIPLES

Jeff G. Konin, MEd, ATC, MPT

OBJECTIVES

After completion of this chapter, the reader will be able to:

DIDACTIC

1. Define Newton's laws of motion.
2. Define a force and list the types of forces that act on the body.
3. Describe how a free body diagram is used to replicate human movement.
4. Explain the role of equilibrium and its importance to human movement.
5. List the types of lever systems that exist and relate their importance to biomechanics.
6. Define mechanical advantage and give an example using the forces of a muscle.
7. Solve equations for muscle and joint forces under situations of equilibrium.

PRACTICAL

1. Explain how Newton's laws of motion apply to human movement.
2. Recognize the various forces that play a role in biomechanics and determine whether each is a facilitator or resistor of movement.
3. Demonstrate how lever systems can be used to modify exercise and activities of daily living.
4. Use mechanical advantage as a component to rehabilitation.
5. Adjust the position of a given resistance to modify muscle force production and joint stress.

INTRODUCTION

As mentioned in the first chapter of this text, the term *biomechanics* refers to the subject of the forces and their effects applied to the total body or to a body link. The study of biomechanics covers two basic areas: statics and dynamics. *Static* biomechanics refers to bodies remaining at rest or in equilibrium as a result of forces acting upon them. *Dynamic* biomechanics refers to the study of moving bodies.

NEWTON'S LAWS

As a way of understanding how a body works with respect to biomechanics, Newton's laws of motion can be used for explanation.[1] Newton's first law is the *law of inertia*. The law of inertia states that a body remains at rest or in uniform motion until acted upon by an unbalanced set of forces. For example, a soccer ball resting on a grass field is in equilibrium since the weight and force of the ball is balanced equally by that of the field. Once the ball is kicked, it will remain in equilibrium and move in a given direction at a given velocity until it is again acted upon by other forces. Forces that can act on the ball in this type of a situation will be discussed later in this chapter. Practically speaking, a force is required to move an object, change its direction or velocity, and to eventually stop the object from moving. Theoretically speaking, an object could not be in equilibrium if only one force is acting upon it. The reason is that there is no other force to counterbalance the original force. This would mean that the object would be in a state other than one of equilibrium. Norkin and Levangie identify some basic principles to follow when considering how forces affect equilibrium:[2]

1. Forces come in pairs.
2. Whenever two solid objects come in contact, they exert a force on each other.
3. Forces on an object are exerted by things that touch that object.
4. Gravity exerts a force on all objects.

Newton's second law is the *law of acceleration*. The law of acceleration states that any change of motion is proportional to the force impressed upon the body, and the direction of change is always in the direction of the force. The law of acceleration takes into account the size of an object, referred to as its *mass*. Using the formula that demonstrates the relationship between acceleration, force, and mass, one can see how this works (a = acceleration; F = force; m = mass of an object):

$$a = F/m$$

Given a fixed mass, a larger force will produce a greater acceleration, and a smaller force will produce a lesser acceleration. If the force was fixed, then the mass of the object will determine the rate of acceleration. For example, with a fixed force, a larger mass will have less acceleration, and a smaller mass will accelerate at a higher rate.

Looking at this principle from a different perspective, consider moving a person who is in a wheelchair or a person who needs to be transferred from one position to another. The heavier the person, that is the more he or she weighs, the greater the force that will be needed to accelerate the movement. This is an important concept that a clinician or therapist must understand. It relates to proper utilization of body mechanics and muscular efficiency.

Newton's third law is the *law of action/reaction*. The law of action/reaction states that whenever two bodies interact, the force of the first body, acting upon the second body, is equal and opposite to the force of the second acting upon the first.[3] In other words, for every action, there is an equal and opposite reaction. Anatomically, this is seen when a person holds a dumbbell weight in the hand. Let us say, for example, that the weight is equal to a force of 5 Newtons. In order for the weight to remain in equilibrium, a force of 5 Newtons must also be counteracting this weight or resistance. In fact, this is actually what happens in this case. In order for the weight to remain in place, a muscle force must be contracting, thus pulling on a bone in a direction opposite that of the weight and equal to the 5 Newtons of the weight (Figure 2-1).

FORCES

To this point, movement and whether or not it is static or dynamic in nature has been briefly discussed. Possibly the most important concept related to human movement is the actual models by which movement is accomplished. These models are referred to in biomechanics as *forces*. A force is simply a push or pull exerted by one object with respect to another object.[4]

A number of different primary forces have commonly been identified in human movement. These include gravity, muscles, externally applied resist-

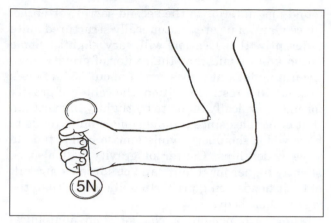

Figure 2-1. Force of the elbow flexor muscle group counterbalancing a 5-Newton weight in the hand.

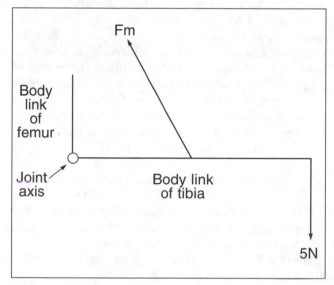

Figure 2-3. Free body diagram.

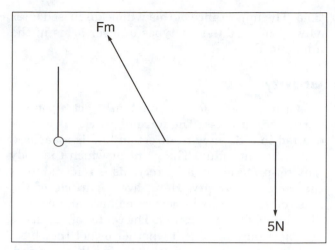

Figure 2-2. Free body diagram of the elbow flexor muscle group and a 5-Newton hand weight.

Free Body Diagrams

When drawing force vectors, a free body diagram is used. This abstract version of human structures simplifies technical illustration and attempts to explain overall forces of objects as they interact with each other. Figure 2-2 demonstrates a free body diagram as a vector force is seen using the previous example of holding a 5-Newton weight in the hand. One can use a free body diagram to accurately assess forces acting upon each other and correlate these findings to clinical application.

Free body diagrams also contain other components. Parts of one's body that are connected by joint articulations are referred to as body links. In the lower extremity, for example, both the femur and the tibia are considered body links. In addition, the joint articulation is referred to as the axis of rotation. This axis of rotation, as seen similarly in measuring range of motion (goniometry), is an imaginary point about which motion occurs (Figure 2-3).

If we were to look at a free body diagram of the tibiofemoral joint that included force vectors representing both the quadriceps and the hamstrings muscle groups, we could label not only the body links and the axis of rotation, but also the point of application of these muscle forces (see Figure 2-3). In this case, the body link can be measured as the distance of a limb. We could also measure the distance from the point of application of a force to the axis of rotation. This measurement is referred to as the *lever arm*. The distance of the lever arm plays a key role in the ability of a force to move an object. The lever arm of the quadriceps muscle distally is very small in comparison to the body link of the

ances, and friction.[5] In biomechanics, a force is described as being a quantity that exhibits both magnitude and direction. That is, the total amount of push or pull is represented by the magnitude, and the course of movement is represented by the direction. Each and every force carries with it similar characteristics that are required by its definition of being a vector quantity. These include having a point of application, a magnitude, and a direction.

A point of application refers to the location where an object is being acted upon. Force vectors are typically represented by straight lines with arrows on one end, indicating the direction of the push or pull. The length of the line, although not always drawn to scale, represents the magnitude of the force that is being exerted.

tibia. The importance of this will be discussed later as we look at different types of lever arms in the human body.

Gravity

Gravitational forces constantly act upon all particles in a mass. The force of gravity is always exerted in a downward direction and is measured as a constant value. The point at which the body may rotate freely in all directions is referred to as the *center of gravity*. Here, every particle of the mass of an object is in perfect balance and equally distributed from the center. The center of gravity of an object plays a role in whether or not the object is in a state of equilibrium. Keeping this in mind, there are three types of equilibrium that apply to this concept: stable, unstable, and neutral.[5]

Stable equilibrium is seen when the center of gravity of an object is displaced, yet the object returns to its original position and so does the center of gravity. This can be seen with a rocking chair. As the chair is pushed, it shifts its center of gravity back and forth a number of times, eventually returning to its original position.

Unstable equilibrium occurs when an object is moved in such a way that its center of gravity is altered and does not return to its original position. While the new position takes on a new identity and a new center of gravity, it is considered unstable with respect to its ability to return to its original state on its own. This is often seen when a person who is simply walking loses his or her balance and falls. The center of gravity shifts immediately. While on the ground, the person may be stable at that point, however, he or she was initially unable to return to the original stable position of standing.

The principle of *neutral equilibrium* is often seen with symmetrically circular objects, such as wheels. With neutral equilibrium, the center of gravity is altered and does not return to its original state. However, it remains at the same level and remains stable throughout its displacement. This is seen most often with a wheelchair. At rest, the chair is stable and the center of gravity is fixed in its original state. If the chair is pushed, it obviously moves, and the center of gravity is displaced with respect to the forces of the ground surface. However, it remains at the same level. The chair will eventually slow down and stop, continuing to be in equilibrium.

In the human body, the center of gravity is found just anterior to the second sacral vertebrae. Since many of us are anatomically structured quite differently, this location will vary slightly. Some authors have said that the center of gravity more accurately falls at a location of about 55% of one's height.[6] In a resting position, the center of gravity for males typically tends to be slightly higher than that of females since a male gender build tends to have wider shoulders, while female builds tend to have wider hips. Center of gravity will also be slightly higher for infants and children as a result of their heads being proportionally larger than the rest of their body.[5]

For each person, a change from anatomical position will result in a change of the center of gravity. Thus, the ability to be able to control one's stability during these changes becomes vitally important during activities of daily living. For example, often times an increase in the lordotic curve of the thoracic spine (forward bending) is seen in a person. This tends to place the center of gravity more anteriorly than normal. Most importantly, it may place the center of gravity too far in front of one's base of support. When standing on two feet, both feet serve as the base of support.

To improve the stability of either static or dynamic equilibrium, the center of gravity should fall within the base of support. Therefore, the larger the base of support, the more stable the position. Likewise, the closer the center of gravity is to the base of support, the more stable the object or person will be. These concepts are well visualized in athletics. First, let's look at a gymnast. Many activities, regardless of event, are performed with the toes of the feet or the fingers of the hands serving as the base of support. This reduces the size of the base of support, making the act of balancing much more difficult.

When the base of support is reduced or narrowed, a smaller amount of force is needed to displace the object or person. Think about a standard kitchen table. Most tables are made with four legs that are actually spread apart from each other underneath the table. This serves as a much more stable base of support as opposed to if the table had one leg underneath the center of it.

The process of using the center of gravity to maximize stability is also seen with the use of assistive devices such as crutches and walkers. Here, these objects are used to widen one's base of support, therefore improving the stability of a person and possibly reducing the risk of a fall.

Friction

Friction, the resistance to relative motion between two bodies in contact, is a force that must be considered when assessing movement. By its nature, a frictional force contains both magnitude and direction. The direction of a frictional force is always opposite in nature to the movement, and it is found in the same plane as the movement. The magnitude of the friction that is encountered varies. However, it is documented as a relative constant value based on the type of surface that is involved with the movement at hand. This is referred to as the *coefficient of friction value*. Typically, the more pliable and rugged a surface is, the higher the coefficient of friction. As the coefficient of friction increases, it means that the forces opposing the movement increase.

When one slides on ice, there is not much of a resistance from the surface. This is because ice has a low coefficient of friction. On the contrary, if one were to slide on artificial grass, the movement would be stopped more suddenly as a result of the rougher surface. In the human body, many anatomical structures will come in contact with one another as movement occurs. Joint surfaces, for example, will be made up, in part, of two or more bones forming an articulation or connecting surface. In healthy bone, these surfaces will glide over one another in a smooth fashion. However, when the outermost surfaces of the bone wear away, such as seen with arthritis, the movement will not be as smooth. The rougher surfaces will lead to increased friction. In turn, this may lead to pain and an ultimate inflammatory response.

Resistance

Resistive forces are always present during movement and must be accounted for. Types of resistive forces range from the actual weight of a limb to any object attached to a body link. Ankle weights, backpacks, and even clothing are all examples of resistive forces. Any object that is being pushed or pulled by a particular muscle or muscle group is also considered a resistive force. Examples of these include doors, furniture, and even exercise machines and equipment. Each type of resistance requires a force of some kind to either counterbalance or overcome it.

FORCES OF A MUSCLE

Each fiber of a muscle contributes to a total force that is exerted by a muscle on a particular bone to which it is attached. The muscle force is recognized as a vector, whereby its point of application is either its proximal or distal attachment. This is determined by which of the two attachments is fixed and which is moving. The point of application is marked at the moving segment of the muscular attachment. The action line, or direction of the vector, is identical to the direction of pull that the muscle is exerting on that bony segment.

Often, more than one force acts on a particular segment. When two or more forces that have a common point of application act on a segment and each of their actions is linear to each other, a *concurrent force* can be determined by simply adding these forces together. The total push or pull, or the sum of these forces, is equal to the concurrent force of the segment. If, for example, a 5-Newton weight is placed on the forearm near the insertion of the main elbow flexors, one could assume that the point of application is nearly the same with respect to a free body diagram. If the elbow flexor muscles exert a force of 7 Newtons in the opposite direction of the weight, then the concurrent force will be 2 Newtons in the direction of the elbow flexor muscle group.

Most movements in the body are not linear in nature, and it therefore becomes slightly more complex to calculate total overall forces. The key here is to again identify all of the forces involved and determine their resultant force. An example of this is seen with the deltoid muscle of the shoulder. This muscle has three components, with each component having the same common distal insertion: the deltoid tuberosity located on the lateral aspect of the humerus approximately one-third of the way down the humerus. Upon contraction, the middle component pulls the humerus directly upward. However, the anterior component pulls the humerus slightly anterior, and the posterior component pulls the humerus slightly posterior, both also pulling in the upward direction. The resultant pull of these three components lies somewhere in the middle (Figure 2-4). If the force of the pull of the anterior component is equal to that of the posterior component, then the resultant direction of pull would be exactly centrally located between the two components. Chapter 3 takes a more detailed look at resultant forces both in linear and nonlinear directions.

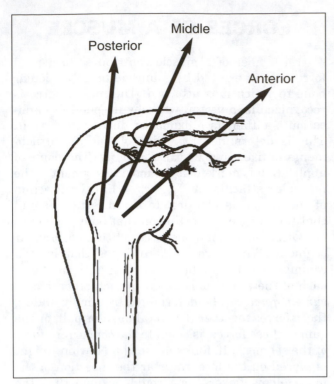

Figure 2-4. Concurrent forces of the deltoid muscle.

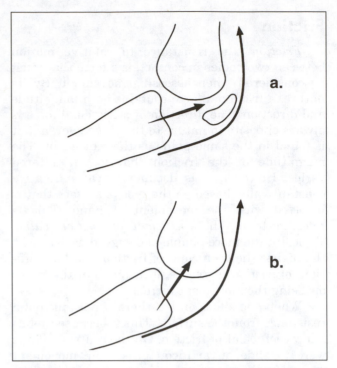

Figure 2-5. Knee extension: a. with a patella; and b. without a patella.

ANATOMICAL PULLEYS

When drawing muscle forces within a free body diagram, the line of action is represented by a vector that resembles a straight line. Rarely in the body do muscles and their fibers actually follow a perfectly straight line. Yet, this principle works well for our purposes of solving biomechanical force-related questions. There are situations that exist in the body in which a muscle actually changes its direction of pull as a result of a reflection of some kind, usually a result of a bony prominence. This is most evident at the knee, where the quadriceps muscle group is diverted by the patella as the common insertion of the four muscles is applied to the tuberosity on the tibia. This aids in changing the overall direction of pull that the muscle exerts. At the knee, for example, without the patella one might have more of a compressive pull in a longitudinal manner. With the presence of the patella allowing for a change of direction, the pull is geared more toward sagittal plane movement, which we know as knee extension (Figure 2-5).

LEVER SYSTEM

A lever is a type of rigid bar that has the ability to rotate around a given axis. In the human body, levers are used to describe body segments as they relate to movement. These segments that the levers represent in the body are the bones. One way of representing and demonstrating movement of the bones is by drawing a lever system.[1,2,5,7,8] A *lever system* has four components:

1. The lever itself, a rigid structure representing the bones of the body
2. A fulcrum, representing a joint axis
3. A force, usually representative of a muscle
4. A resistance, a force that must be overcome by a muscle

It is not uncommon for a lever system to contain more than one force or resistance. In fact, most complex systems that are represented in the body contain just that. The purpose of using a lever system to represent a movement of a body link is for the purpose of identifying all aspects of movement related to the particular structure. One must

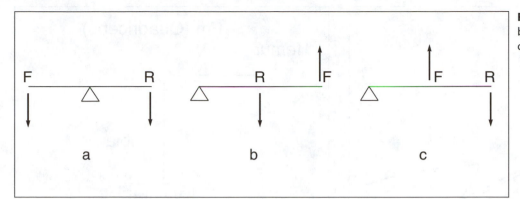

Figure 2-6. Levers of the body: a. first class; b. second class; and c. third class.

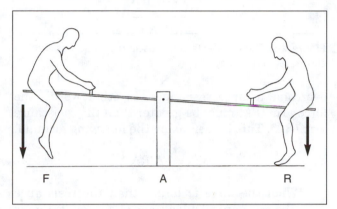

Figure 2-7. Example of a first-class lever is a seesaw.

remember that the body itself is comprised of a number of lever systems that are linked together.

There are primarily three types of levers that exist, while some are found more commonly than others in the human body. These are called first-, second-, and third-class levers.

Both the muscle forces and the resistance forces act to influence the overall movement of a lever. Since the movement occurs about an axis of rotation, movement will be performed either in a clockwise or counterclockwise direction depending on which force is stronger. In addition, the distance between the forces and the axis of rotation plays an important role in the determining movement. This distance is referred to as the force arm and the resistance arm, respectively.

First-Class Levers

A *first-class lever* is described as having the fulcrum in between the muscle force and the resistance force, while both of these forces are acting in opposite rotational directions (Figure 2-6). This type of a lever is primarily designed for balance. A classic example of a first-class lever is a see-saw. If a child is sitting on either end, each would represent a force on one side of the fulcrum. Depending

on the weight of each child and the distance each is from the fulcrum, the seesaw would either be in balance or it would rotate in one direction (Figure 2-7).

In the human body, very few first-class levers exist. One example that does exist is seen in the vertebral column. While one attempts to hold his or her body upright using the erector spinae muscle group, the force of gravity is attempting to forwardly bend the vertebral column. The ability of the person to use the posterior muscles of the spine to counteract the forces of gravity will determine whether or not this person will be able to stand up straight in a vertically balanced position.

Second-Class Levers

Second-class levers are designed much differently than first-class levers. With second-class levers, both the force arm and the resistance arm are on the same side of the fulcrum. Not only are the forces acting in opposite directions, but the force arm of the muscle is greater than the resistance arm (see Figure 2-6). This type of a configuration is specifically designed for power. That is, since the force arm of the muscle is greater than the resistance arm, one would expect that a smaller force is needed to move a given resistance. In the human body, it is arguable whether or not any true second-class levers actually exist. A common piece of equipment that is used to explain how a second-class lever works is the wheelbarrow. With a wheelbarrow, the resistance is located closer to the fulcrum, while the muscle forces act in the opposite direction, utilizing a longer force arm (Figure 2-8).

Third-Class Levers

Most lever systems in the body are of the *third-class lever* type. Here again, the resistance and the muscle force act in opposite directions. However,

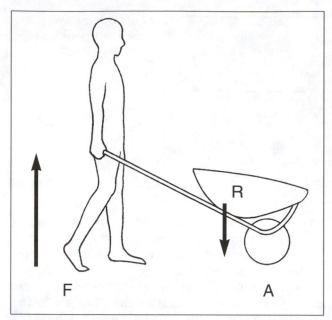

Figure 2-8. A wheelbarrow is an example of a second-class lever.

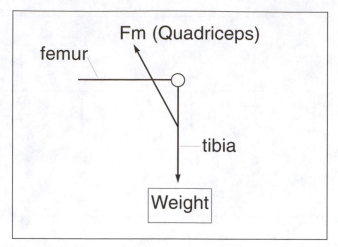

Figure 2-9. The knee extensor muscle group acts as a third-class lever in the body.

the lever arm of the muscle force is shorter than the lever arm of the resistance (see Figure 2-6). This set-up is not designed for power, but instead is at a disadvantage to move a given resistance. In other words, more force is required to move a given resistance. One advantage of third-class levers is that they are designed for producing range of motion and speed. This is accomplished since a relatively small amount of muscle shortening is needed to gain rotational movement around a joint axis.

In the human body, third-class levers are seen quite often. This is because most muscles attach near joint articulations or close to the axis of rotation. This is seen, for example, at the knee when looking at the quadriceps muscle group (Figure 2-9). Together, the muscle group inserts at the tibial tubercle, just beyond the tibiofemoral joint. In addition to the resistance of gravity, when one moves into a position of knee extension, most resistive forces, such as ankle weights, are located more distally along the tibia. Therefore, while a small contractile shortening of the muscle is needed to produce range of motion changes, a larger effort is required to actually overcome any resistance that is located further down the leg.

MECHANICAL ADVANTAGE

The term *mechanical advantage* (MA) refers to the efficiency of a lever. A lever is considered to be efficient only when a small effort is required to overcome a large resistance. In other words, the force arm (FA) must be greater than the resistance arm (RA). This is seen using the following formula:

$$MA = FA/RA$$

When the force is larger than the resistance arm, the mechanical advantage of a lever system is greater than one. The larger the number, the more efficient the lever and the better chance it has to produce power. In a second-class lever in which the force arm is always greater than the resistance arm, systems are inherently at a mechanical advantage. This is not true in third-class levers in which the resistance arm is always greater than the force arm. In third-class levers, the mechanical advantage will always be less than one, and is considered to be at a mechanical disadvantage, or inefficient. First-class levers can be either mechanically advantageous or disadvantageous depending on which arm, the force or the resistance, is closer to the resistance.

Clinical Relevance of Mechanical Advantage

Since most muscles in the body work from a mechanically disadvantageous set-up, a clinician must be creative in designing exercises and activities that do not further predispose one to difficult and potentially dangerous situations. This said, there are ways of modifying various exercises and activities to enhance one's ability to perform in a more efficient manner.

To better explain this principle, let us examine an individual who has recently undergone arthro-

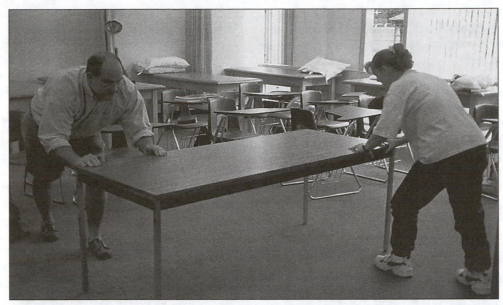

Figure 2-10. Example of a table being moved in opposite directions by two people. This demonstrates the principle of a force couple.

scopic knee surgery. Let us assume that you have instructed this person to do three sets of 10 repetitions each of a seated knee extension exercise using a 2-pound weight as a resistance. The person reports significant difficulty in performing the activity you have requested. You also notice that the person is unable to perform the exercise through a complete range of motion. This leaves you with a decision-making process.

Naturally, there are a number of ideas that come to mind. First, you can reduce the number of sets or even repetitions. While this may be effective, it will not enable the individual to perform the task by moving through a greater range of motion. The next logical step might be to reduce the weight of the resistance. This is a good idea and can be easily done. Using biomechanical principles, there are some other alternatives that can also be used. The position of the exercise can be modified. That is, instead of performing the knee extension from a sitting position, one could attempt to perform the exercise from a side-lying position. This position change would reduce the effect of gravity as a resistive force. While this is not truly considered to be a "gravity eliminated" position, it can be considered a "gravity reduced" position.

The seated knee extension exercise is performed primarily through a third-class lever, as discussed earlier. This means that the resistance of the weight is located further from the fulcrum, in this case the knee joint, than the insertion of the quadriceps muscle group. While the type of lever

cannot be changed and still allow for the same exercise to be performed, it is very feasible to reposition the weight more proximally on the tibia so that the resistance arm is reduced. This in turn will not require as much of a muscle force to overcome the weight and may consequently allow for the individual to now complete a greater range of motion using the same resistance.

The process of altering exercise and activity by using the principles of mechanical advantage not only allows one to perform exercises with a higher success rate, but also reduces the risk of potential injury and helps to psychologically motivate an individual through the completion of an act that may not have otherwise been successfully performed.

FORCE COUPLES

Body muscles have the ability to work individually or together to produce movement. Earlier, we discussed the concept of concurrent forces, in which different muscles can contract to perform a resultant movement. Similar to this principle is that of a *force couple*. A force couple is defined as muscles working in opposite directions to accomplish a similar motion. This is seen most clearly with movement of the scapula, whereas a contraction of the upper trapezius results in lateral rotation of the scapula. The fibers of the upper trapezius move in a superior direction when this occurs. When the lower trapezius fibers contract, the scapula also moves in a laterally rotated direction. However, the fibers of the lower trapezius move inferiorly. Both sections of fibers, while moving in opposite directions, contribute to the same movement.

The classic example used to describe a force couple in its purest form is when one attempts to perform a rotational movement of a large object such as a piece of furniture. To accomplish rotation in the same direction, it is possible that one person can pull the object in one direction while another person pulls the object in the opposite direction (Figure 2-10).

EQUILIBRIUM EQUATIONS

Determining whether or not an object is in fact in equilibrium involves a step-by-step process that examines all of the forces that are acting on the object. This is done by utilizing free body diagrams and placing these forces into mathematical equations. Three conditions must exist for a body or object to be in static equilibrium:

- The sum of all vertical forces must equal zero
- The sum of all horizontal forces must equal zero
- The sum of all the rotational forces must equal zero

$$\Sigma F_V = 0$$
$$\Sigma F_H = 0$$
$$\Sigma F_T = 0$$

We have already discussed the possibility of forces such as gravity, friction, and muscle pull having an effect on movement. It is important to be able to distinguish the direction which the movement is occurring, that is, vertically, horizontally, or rotationally. Gravity, for example, occurs in a downward or inferiorly vertical direction. Muscle actions can create vertical, horizontal, and even rotational directional forces. Rotational forces are more commonly known as *torques* and involve not only the force of the muscle but also the distance of the moment arm of that particular muscle. Therefore, a torque or rotational force is the product of a force times its perpendicular distance from its line of action to the axis of motion (moment arm).

When solving for equilibrium, it is not possible to use terms such as superior, inferior, left, right, clockwise, or counterclockwise within equations. Therefore, these directional terms are given values with respect to positive (+) and negative (-). For example, upward vertical forces are often referred to as being numerically positive (+), while downward forces are negative (-). Similarly, horizontal forces to the left are considered negative (-) and those to the right are positive (+). Torques in a clockwise direction are considered positive (+), while those in a counterclockwise direction are referred to as negative (-). While it is not critically important if one were to reverse these symbols, it is imperative that they remain constant throughout the entire equation-solving process. That is, one could easily call a clockwise movement a negative (-) movement as long as all clockwise movements are referred to as negative (-) movements throughout the remainder of the equation. The importance of this will be demonstrated in the following examples. Identifying the direction of forces is one of a number of steps that will help to correctly solve equilibrium equations (Table 2-1).

Strategies to Solve Equilibrium Problems

Let us look at a situation in which a first-class lever is in static equilibrium. In this particular equation, both the lever arm distances and the forces acting upon the axis of rotation will be given. We will solve for the force that is acting upon the axis of rotation.

Therefore:

Question: Assuming this system is in equilibrium, what is the force acting upon the fulcrum?

Given:

- Force A = 10 Newtons (N)
- Force B = 15 N
- Force A distance from fulcrum = 3 meters (m)
- Force B distance from fulcrum = 2 m

To solve for the force at the fulcrum we must incorporate the formulas of the forces acting on this system. Let us first look at the horizontal forces. The sum of the horizontal forces must equal zero. However, in this particular system, no horizontal forces are identified. Therefore, it is safe to assume that the forces are already equal.

Next we can look at the vertical forces. Again, the sum of all vertical forces must equal zero. The two vertical forces we encounter are that of Force A and Force B. Notice both are in a downward direction and, as a result, are labeled in a negative

(-) fashion:

$$\Sigma V_F = 0 = (-10 \text{ N}) + (-15 \text{ N})$$

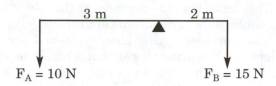

Remember, we are looking to identify the force of the fulcrum. This must be reflected in the equation. Since we are told that the system is in equilibrium, we know that the force of the fulcrum must be able to counteract that of the sum of Force A and Force B. This means that the force of the fulcrum must be labeled positive (+):

$$(-10 \text{ N}) + (- 15 \text{ N}) + F_f = 0$$

Solving this equation, we find:

$$(-10 \text{ N}) - 15 \text{ N} + F_f = 0$$

whereas:

$$-25 \text{ N} + F_f = 0$$

whereas:

$$F_f = 25 \text{ N}$$

Since 25 N is a positive (+) force, this tells us that the force of the fulcrum is acting in the upward or superior direction. Remember, a negative number in these equations does not represent a negative value of a force. It simply means that a force is acting in a downward direction.

One more step that we should take is to verify that the system is, in fact, in equilibrium. This is done by solving for all of the rotational forces, or the torques:

$$\Sigma T = 0$$

From the given system, we find a force that can potentially rotate this system in a clockwise (+) direction (Force B) as well as a force that can rotate this system in a counterclockwise (-) direction (Force A). Solving for rotational equilibrium then involves these forces multiplied by each of their moment arms and added together to equal 0. Because each of these forces is perpendicular to the lever arm, the lever arm, and the moment arm are equivalent in value. If, however, these were not perpendicular, trigonometric formulas would need to be utilized to calculate the moment of the forces (Appendix B).

Solving for rotational equilibrium:

$$(-10 \text{ N})(3 \text{ m}) + (15 \text{ N}) (2 \text{ m}) = 0$$

where:

$$(-30 \text{ Nm}) + (30 \text{ Nm}) = 0$$
$$\text{and: } 0 = 0$$

Since one force is moving the object 30 Nm in a clockwise direction and the other force is moving the object 30 Nm in a counterclockwise direction as well, the object is therefore in rotational equilibrium.

Let us examine another example of a system that is in static equilibrium.

Question: What is the force of the elbow flexor muscle when holding a 5 N weight around the wrist? What is the force that is acting at the elbow joint?

Given: weight = 5 N
- lever arm of weight = 30 cm
- lever arm of muscle = 10 cm
- angle of elbow flexion = 90°

Here is what the free body diagram of the equation should look like:

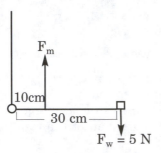

Again, in this situation, the force of gravity has already been accounted for in the force of the weight and the muscle. When labeling the force of the joint (F), there is no way of knowing in advance whether or not the force will be in an upward or downward direction. A positive value is usually given to the force in this type of situation in an attempt to simplify calculations. Also, because the elbow joint is at 90°, the moment arm is the same value as the lever arm.

Once again, in this example we do not see any horizontal forces, so we can assume the sum of the horizontal forces is already at zero. Next, we need to decide if we should solve for the unknown muscle force or the joint force. Looking at the equation, we can see that if we choose to solve for the joint force we would need to use an equation that would solve for the sum of all vertical forces. This equation would look like this:

$$\Sigma F_v = F_j + F_m + (-5 \text{ N}) = 0$$

Because there are two unknowns—the force of the joint and the force of the muscle—this equation cannot be solved at this time. Let us then look at the sum of the rotational forces:

$$(-5 \text{ N}) (30 \text{ cm}) + (F_m)(10 \text{ cm}) + (F_j) (0) = 0$$

This can be solved even though there are again two unknowns. The reason is the joint force is at the axis of rotation, indicating it is 0 distance away

and therefore has no moment arm. So, when calculating, it will cancel itself out as being a rotational force. Solving this equation, we find:

$$(-150 \text{ Ncm}) + (F_m \ 10 \text{ cm}) = 0$$
$$F_m \ 10 \text{ cm} = 150 \text{ Ncm}$$
$$F_m = 15 \text{ N}$$

The force of the muscle equals 15 N in an upward direction. Knowing this, we can substitute this value in the equation for vertical forces and now solve for the force of the joint:

$$F_j + 15 \text{ N} + (-5 \text{ N}) = 0$$
$$F_j + 15 \text{ N} - 5 \text{ N} = 0$$
$$F_j + 10 \text{ N} = 0$$
$$F_j = -10 \text{ N}$$

This indicates that the force at the elbow joint is equal to 10 N in the downward direction.

The purpose of this chapter is to help one understand the principles of biomechanics as they apply to everyday practice. Considering the situation discussed earlier in which an individual was having difficulty overcoming a certain resistance, let us now examine the effect that moving the weight closer to the joint axis has on the muscle force required to keep the elbow at 90° and the ultimate effect on joint forces.

Using the same conditions, we will now say that the weight is located 20 cm from the joint axis instead of 30 cm. Solving for rotational forces:

$$(F_m) (10 \text{ cm}) + (-5 \text{ N}) (20 \text{ cm}) + (F_j) (0) = 0$$
$$F_m \ 10 \text{ cm} - 100 \text{ Ncm} = 0$$
$$F_m \ 10 \text{ cm} = 100 \text{ Ncm}$$
$$F_m = 10 \text{ N}$$

The force required of the muscle to now lift the weight and keep the elbow at a 90° angle has been reduced from 15 N to 10 N. This allows for an individual to use a lesser effort when attempting to lift the resistance. A situation of this kind can benefit one who has muscle atrophy as a result of an injury or surgery, or for an individual who has accompanied pain with increased muscular effort. What effect does this have on the elbow joint force? To determine this, we must use the equation to solve for vertical forces:

$$F_j + 10 \text{ N} + (-5 \text{ N}) = 0$$
$$F_j + 10 \text{ N} - 5 \text{ N} = 0$$
$$F_j + 5 \text{ N} = 0$$
$$F_j = -5 \text{ N}$$

What we see is that the force at the joint has reduced from 10 N to 5 N in the same direction. In this example, simply moving the resistance one-third of the distance closer to the joint axis has resulted in reducing the joint forces by one-half. Again, clinically, this has significant impact. By keeping the resistance constant, a clinician can reduce the forces at a joint or control the amount of muscle force required to counteract a given resistance by simply changing the moment arm.

The ability to accommodate a person who is having difficulty in performing a task that requires overcoming resistance is a powerful tool that a clinician can use to aid in the rehabilitation process. However, these principles can also be used to enhance the performance of a muscle by requiring it to use a greater force to move a resistance. For example, assume you are given the task of designing a home exercise program for a person who has a set of sand weights. The heaviest weight this person owns is 3 pounds. If lifting the 3-pound sand weight is not challenging enough for the person, you could have this person move the weight to a position that is more distal from the joint axis in an attempt to increase the muscle force required to move the weight. Biomechanically, you are simply increasing the moment arm of the weight. When increasing the moment arm for intentions such as increasing the functional capacity of a muscle to forcefully contract, you must be aware of the effects that the exercise will have on related joint surfaces. It is a challenge for the practicing clinician to balance the risks and benefits of muscular output versus joint stresses that accompany the changes associated with altering and modifying physical activity and rehabilitative exercises.

References

1. Rasch PJ. *Kinesiology and Applied Anatomy.* 7th ed. Philadelphia, Pa: Lea & Febiger; 1989.
2. Norkin C, Levangie P. *Joint Structure and Function: A Comprehensive Analysis.* Philadelphia, Pa: FA Davis Company; 1988.
3. Cromer AH. *Physics for Life Sciences.* 2nd ed. New York, NY: McGraw Hill; 1977.
4. *Webster's Ninth New Collegiate Dictionary.* Springfield, Mass: Merriam-Webster, Inc; 1984.
5. Lehmkuhl LD, Smith LK. *Brunnstrom's Clinical Kinesiology.* 4th ed. Philadelphia, Pa: FA Davis Company; 1983.
6. Hellebrandt FA. Location of the cardinal anatomical orientation planes passing through the center of weight in young adult women. *Am J Physiol.* 1938; 121:465.
7. Soderberg GL. *Kinesiology: Application to Pathological Motion.* Baltimore, Md: Williams & Wilkins; 1986.
8. Lippert LA. *Clinical Kinesiology for Physical Therapist Assistants.* 2nd ed. Philadelphia, Pa: FA Davis Company; 1994.

Suggested Reading

Basmajian JV. *Muscles Alive.* 4th ed. Baltimore, Md: Williams & Wilkins; 1978.

Frankel VH, Nordin M. *Basic Biomechanics of the Skeletal System.* Philadelphia, Pa: Lea & Febiger; 1980.

Kapandji IA. *The Physiology of Joints, Vol 1, Upper Limb.* London: E & S Livingstone; 1970.

Kapandji IA. *The Physiology of Joints, Vol 2, Lower Limb.* London: E & S Livingstone; 1970.

Kapandji IA. *The Physiology of the Joints, Vol 3, The Trunk and Vertebral Column.* Edinborough: Churchill Livingstone; 1974.

Schenck JM, Cordova FD. *Introductory Biomechanics.* 2nd ed. Philadelphia, Pa: FA Davis Company; 1980.

White AA, Punjabi MM. *Clinical Biomechanics of the Spine.* Philadelphia, Pa: JB Lippincott; 1978.

1. List each of Newton's laws of motion. Define each and give an example of how they work with respect to the human body.

2. Define a force. What are the various types of forces that act on the body?

3. How does a free body diagram help in understanding biomechanics? What are the components of a free body diagram?

4. How can gravity be reduced when performing an activity?

5. What is the difference between stable, unstable, and neutral equilibrium? Give an example of each.

6. If you were to carry a couple of books under your left arm, would this change your center of gravity? What about if the books were held across your chest? Would the center of gravity change if you had the books in a knapsack carried on your back?

7. How does the base of support differ for each of the following scenarios:
   a. Standing in anatomical position
   b. Standing on one leg
   c. Standing on one leg with the aid of two crutches (one on each side)
   d. In a quadruped position (on hands and knees)
   e. On the toes of one foot
   f. Sitting in a chair

8. How does friction affect joint surfaces in the body?

9. List the components of a lever system. How does the location of the forces affect mechanical advantage?

10. How can you as a clinician use lever systems to assist you during the rehabilitation process?

11. Estimate the force at the fulcrum during equilibrium conditions for the following two children sitting on a seesaw. How can you be assured that the seesaw is, in fact, in rotational equilibrium?
    Child A weighs 10 kg and is located 2 m away from the fulcrum.
    Child B weighs 20 kg and is on the other end 1 m away from the fulcrum.

12. Estimate the muscle force of the hamstring muscle group and the joint stress occurring at the knee under the following equilibrium conditions. How much muscle force would be required to keep the knee flexed to 90° if the weight were located 30 cm from the knee joint? What effect would this have on the force acting upon the knee joint?
    Knee angle = 90° of flexion
    Weight at ankle = 5 kg
    Lever arm of weight = 40 cm
    Lever arm of muscle = 10 cm

CHAPTER 3

JOINT STRUCTURE AND FUNCTION

Jeff G. Konin, MEd, ATC, MPT

OBJECTIVES

After completion of this chapter, the reader will be able to:

DIDACTIC

1. Identify common structures of bone and become familiar with their functions.
2. Identify common structures associated with the make-up of joints and become familiar with their functions.
3. Recognize the classification systems used to identify the types of joints.
4. List the types of receptors associated with joints.
5. Compare compression, tension, bending, torsion, and shear as they relate to joint function.
6. Define stress and strain.
7. Compare arthrokinematics and arthrokinetics.
8. Understand the role of rotary and translatory motion within a joint.
9. Explain the convex-concave rule and its relationship to joint movement.
10. Describe the effects of joint deformation.

PRACTICAL

1. Palpate various bones and joints within the body.
2. Perform joint movements that incorporate compression, tension, bending, torsion, and shear.
3. Demonstrate the convex-concave rule using a skeletal model.
4. Using a skeletal model, identify joints that possess rotary and translatory motion.

STRUCTURE OF BONE

Tissue can be defined as an organized group of cells that are similar in appearance and function.[1] In the human body, there are four major types of tissue: epithelial, connective, muscle, and nervous.

Bone is considered to be the hardest of connective tissues within the body. It is comprised of a matrix that contains many minerals. In general, the outer surface of the bone is referred to as *cortical* and is said to be slightly stronger than the spongy or inner portion of the bone. *Spongy* bone lies within *compact* bone and contains many of the nutrients used for the development of red blood cells. Age, sex, and other elements of one's physiology may influence the material properties of a bone.[2] Furthermore, the strength of a bone may be enhanced through a process called *adaptive remodeling*, whereby stresses and strains to a bone increase the ability of that particular structure to remain in continuity. There are limits to the amount of stress and strain that a bone can withstand—too much may lead to breakdown and result in a fracture. This can be seen with prolonged time spent in abnormal postures, as bone can atrophy and eventually breakdown. Osteoporosis, for example, is an age-related disorder characterized by a decrease in bone mass. Without proper nutrition and adequate strengthening of the bone, women more so than men are at risk for fracture with this condition.[3] Intervening with normal muscular activity can provide bones with the ability to carry a greater load and absorb more energy before breakdown can occur.[4]

Surrounding the outer surface of the bone is another form of connective tissue referred to as *hyaline cartilage*. This silky, smooth covering possesses a glass-like appearance and serves primarily to protect the articulating surfaces of the bone.[5-7]

Bones have historically been referred to as being either long, short, flat, or irregular in nature. *Long bones*, typically found in the limbs, are designed for weightbearing and spatial movements. They frequently serve as distal muscle attachments and create various pulley-like effects, as described in Chapter 2. *Short bones* are rather small and cubical in shape. These are found in the hands and feet, represented by the carpals and tarsals, respectively. Short bones contain strong interconnective ligamentous support and function both to allow for mobility and to assist with stability. As will be demonstrated later, the tarsal bones of the foot must be able to adapt to many different surfaces during weightbearing activity and therefore play a diverse role between flexibility and rigidity.[8]

Flat bones, like long bones, also contain many muscular attachments. However, unlike long bones that connect with muscles, in many cases via long extensive tendons, flat bones are more broad in nature and allow for a larger area of surface for muscular attachment. The sternum, scapulae, and ilium are examples of flat bones. *Irregular bones* do not fall into a single classification, but instead are rather different even from one another. The pubis, the maxilla, and the bodies of the vertebrae are examples of irregular bones.[8]

STRUCTURE OF JOINTS

When two or more bones come together at a similar location, a *joint* or *articulation* is formed. Articulations of bones come in many forms, but in general serve to accomplish one of two functions: mobility or stability of a joint. The relationship between mobility and stability at any joint within the human body is one of an inverse nature. That is, a joint that provides for much mobility is likely to be more unstable. Likewise, a joint that is not very mobile is usually found to be more stable. This will be demonstrated throughout the text as each particular joint is more closely examined. In addition, one will notice that a joint that is primarily designed for stability purposes will in general contain less complex structures, whereas a joint that functions to allow multiple movements will contain many more complex structures, allowing for greater ranges of motion throughout multiple planes. It should be made clear that most joints within the body contribute to both mobility and stability simultaneously, to varying degrees.

Norkin and Levangie identify four simple principles that can be followed with respect to the structure of a joint:[9]

1. The design of a joint is constructed by its function and the nature of the components.
2. Once a joint is constructed, the structures of a joint will determine its function.
3. Joints that serve a single function are less complex than joints that serve multiple functions.
4. Joints designed primarily for stability are less complex than joints designed primarily for mobility.

Table 3-1
Structures Involved in Joint Articulation

Bone: connective tissue forming an articulation.
Hyaline cartilage: clear, glossy covering that protects the ends of bone.
Fibrocartilage: tougher cartilage containing elastic properties allowing for accommodation of pressure, friction, and shear forces at articulating surfaces, also referred to as menisci.
Synovial fluid: thick, clear fluid that lubricates a joint, allowing for less resistance to joint motion, also helps to nourish cartilaginous structures.
Ligaments: dense connective tissue connecting bone to bone, providing for stability.
Tendons: elastic connective tissue connecting muscle to bone that assists with joint movement.
Muscle: connective tissue that contracts to create movement about a joint, as well as assist with stability of a joint.

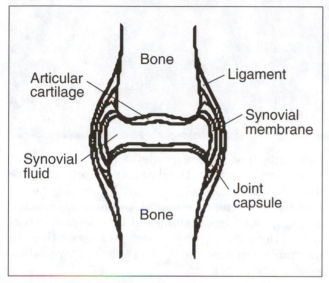

Figure 3-1. Joint capsule.

There are a number of anatomical materials used to assist with the articulation of a joint. Each of these structures serves a unique purpose and plays an important role with respect to its contribution to the mobility and stability of a joint. Table 3-1 lists these structures and briefly explains their roles.

Joints that contain copious amounts of synovial fluid are surrounded by a joint capsule. This joint capsule serves primarily to protect the articular surfaces of the bones that comprise the joint. The capsule consists of two distinct layers, the *stratum fibrosum* and the *stratum synovium*. The stratum fibrosum is the outer layer of the capsule. It is made of fibrous tissue and provides support and protection to the joint. In many cases, ligaments to surrounding joints may blend with this portion of the capsule to reinforce the stability of the joint. The stratum synovium is the inner layer.

It is lined with a synovial membrane that is comprised of thick, vascular connective tissue. The main function of this layer is to secrete synovial fluid. The viscosity of this fluid varies inversely with the joint velocity or rate of shear. That is, when the bony components of a joint are moving rapidly, the viscosity of the fluid decreases and provides less resistance to motion (Figure 3-1).

Joint Classification

Joints are classified in a number of ways that help to identify the function of a particular joint. The three major classes are:

1. synarthrodial, or immovable;
2. amphiarthrodial, or slightly movable
3. diarthrodial, or freely movable.

It is not uncommon to recognize overlapping of this classification system within the literature, as some authors do not agree as to the exact representation of each joint.[8-12] Table 3-2 illustrates a more descriptive breakdown of these classifications.

A *synarthrotic* or immovable joint is primarily a direct union of two or more bones via dense fibrous tissue. Three types that have been identified are the suture, gomphosis, and syndesmosis. These can be found in the areas of the body such as the coronal suture, a tooth, and the distal radioulnar joint, respectively.

Amphiarthrotic joints represent unions formed by fibrocartilage or hyaline cartilage. The two main types are a symphysis and a synchondrosis. Examples of these types of joints are found in the pubic symphysis and first sternocostal joint, respectively.

Diarthrodial joints are designed for movement and typically surrounded by synovial capsules.

Table 3-2
Classification of Joints

Major Class	Type	Example	Connective Method
Synarthrotic	1. Suture	1. Coronal suture	Dense fibrous tissue
	2. Gomphosis	2. Tooth	
	3. Syndesmosis	3. DRUJ	
Amphiarthrotic	1. Symphysis	1. Pubic symphysis	Cartilage
	2. Synchondrosis	2. First sternocostal joint	
Diarthrodial	Uniaxial		
	1a. Hinge	1a. Interphalangeals	1. Capsule
	1b. Pivot	1b. Atlanto-axial joint	2. Synovial fluid
			3. Menisci
	Biaxial		
	2a. Condyloid	2a. MP joint	
	2b. Saddle	2b. CMC joint	
	Triaxial		
	3a. Plane joint	3a. Carpals	
	3b. Ball-and-socket	3b. Hip	

These joints have been classically labeled as being uniaxial, biaxial, or triaxial. As synovial type joints, the union of the articulation may be influenced by such structures as the capsule, synovial fluid, and menisci, among others. Table 3-2 lists examples of the types of diarthrodial joints within the human body.

Joint Receptors

Each joint contains receptors that enable one to perceive change in a specific joint. Depending on the type of receptor that is contained and activated, a joint may be sensitive to change via different mechanisms. *Ruffini nerve endings* and *Pacinian corpuscles* are both examples of receptors that can be found within the outer layers of a joint capsule. Ruffini nerve endings are represented with higher concentrations in proximal joints and are sensitive to stretching of a joint capsule, changes in joint position, and changes in synovial pressure within a joint. Pacinian corpuscles, on the other hand, are found in higher concentrations in distal joints and more commonly respond to high-frequency vibration and high-velocity changes with respect to the position of a joint. These have been described as responding to deep pressures resulting from body tissue deformation.[5-8,13]

Golgi ligament endings are receptors located in ligaments that form articulations. These respond to a stretch within the ligament itself and are found in essentially all joints, with the exception of those comprising the spinal column. *Free nerve endings*, found in capsular and ligamentous structures throughout the body, are sensitive to mechanical stresses and external or internal biomechanical stimuli.[5-8,13]

JOINT FUNCTION

As mentioned earlier, joints play a role in mobility and stability. This is facilitated by the properties of the tissues that comprise the joint and the forces that are applied to a joint at a given time. Many pathological conditions, including but not limited to degenerative joint disease and adhesive capsulitis, are greatly affected by these varying forces. While all of these forces can become extensive and lead to tissue damage, they are, in fact, normal components of joint function, as they must occur in order for the articular surfaces to function in an optimal manner.

The relaxed or resting position of a joint that has no forces being applied to it is referred to as being *unloaded*. If joints were to remain unloaded at all times, they would not undergo the desired amount of stresses to enable them to become

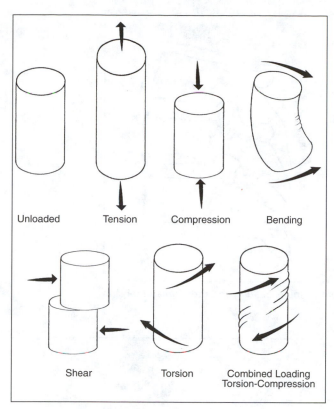

Figure 3-2. Types of joint forces.

stronger. Therefore, forces must be applied to periodically *load* these joints (Figure 3-2). The following are types of forces commonly seen acting on joint surfaces:

Compression: the act of pressing together, in which the space between the articulating bones is decreased proportionally in the same plane.

Tension: the normal force that tends to stretch or pull bones apart from one another. Here, the joint space is increased.

Bending: also referred to as deformation, in which a load is applied to an area where there is not direct support, thus creating a curved-type compression. Here, joint space will decrease on one side of the articulation while it will increase on the other.

Torsion: the force that tends to twist a body, in which the rotation occurs in one direction to a bone and in the opposite direction to its articulating bone.

Shear: a horizontal force that is applied parallel to the joint surface as in a scraping motion between the articulating bones.

APPLICATIONS OF JOINT FORCES

It is clear that joints do not remain dormant and must rely on intermittent acceptable forces over time so that they can continue to function in a desirable manner. These forces can also be referred to as stresses. *Stress* within a joint is the resistance of a body to the deforming actions of an outside force. So, a stress is simply the action of change to a joint. The measurement of this deformation is identified as the strain. Therefore, *strain* describes the changes in the dimensions of a body as a result of an applied load.[12,14]

Many joints of the spine and lower extremities are constantly stressed via compressional forces during standing and weightbearing activities throughout one's normal daily activities. In addition, muscles have the ability to create degrees of strain when they contract either through tension or compression.

When one bends at the spine, again compression and tension can be witnessed. With forward bending, compression occurs to the anterior aspect of the vertebral joints while simultaneous tension occurs to the posterior aspect. The reverse can be seen with backward bending (Figure 3-3). Rotation of the trunk not only creates torsional forces among the intervertebral joints, but also has the potential to create shear forces if the intervertebral joints are in a position of compression (Figure 3-4). Each of these stresses has the ability to increase in direct proportion to the amount of distance that is moved.

KINEMATICS

Joints within the human body are said to fall within a *kinematic chain*. A kinematic chain refers to a series of links that are interconnected by a series of joints. This means that one link at one joint will produce motion at all other joints within the system in a predictable manner.

These kinematic chains are said to act in either an open or closed position. A *closed kinematic chain* is one in which the distal extremity is fixed on the ground or to an object. For example, when standing, one has both feet weightbearing on the ground. Since the feet, serving as the distal portion

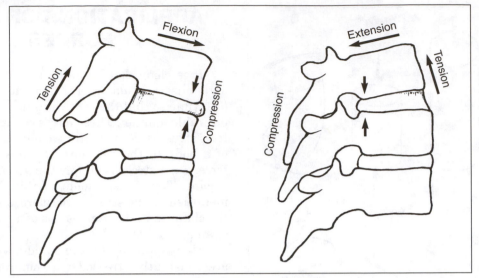

Figure 3-3. Forward and backward bending of the spine creating compression and tension simultaneously.

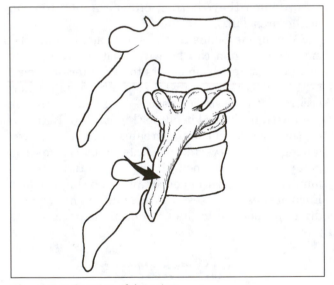

Figure 3-4. Rotation of the spine.

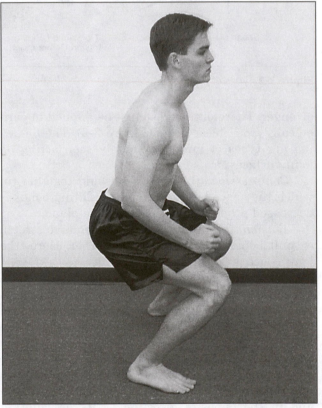

Figure 3-5. Closed kinematic position of the lower extremity.

of the chain, are fixated to the ground, the person is said to be in a closed kinematic position with respect to the lower extremity (Figure 3-5). By contrast, the same person who is standing may motion with the wrist in a wave-like fashion. Since the wrist is not fixated to an object, it can function and move without actually creating any predictable movement at the elbow or shoulder joints. This is referred to as an *open kinematic chain*. While these examples may be relatively simple to comprehend, human movement can be quite complex. For example, when one ambulates, the lower extremities constantly vary with respect to being in an open versus closed kinematic chain position.

Arthrokinematics vs. Arthrokinetics

The movement of a single bone is referred to as *osteokinematic motion*. This movement, combined with the movement or stationary position of an adjacent bone, creates movement about a joint that

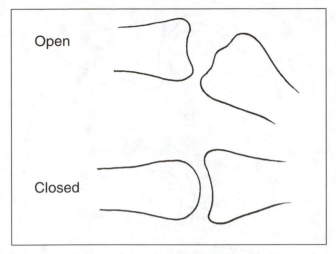

Figure 3-6. Open and closed packed positions of a joint.

is referred to as *arthrokinematics*. While arthrokinematics explains movement of a joint with respect to time, it does not necessarily take into account the reasons for such movement, which may include force and momentum. It does include such factors as displacement, velocity, and acceleration that may influence the rate of movement.

Available anatomical or physiological range of motion varies from joint to joint. These ranges vary depending on the surrounding structures of each joint, including surface areas, capsular extensibility, and musculotendinous flexibility, to name a few. Within the anatomical range of each joint, positions exist that are referred to as either loose or taut.

When the surfaces of a joint are maximally congruent and the surrounding capsuloligamentous structures are maximally taut, the joint is said to be in a *closed packed* or *locked* position. In this position, the joint is said to be most stable with respect to distractional type forces. By contrast, when a joint is in a position whereby the bony surfaces move relatively free upon one another and the surrounding capsuloligamentous structures are relatively slack, it is said to be in a *loose packed, open packed,* or *unlocked* position. While joints may possess a position in which the structures are the most slack, essentially any position away from the fully locked position can be considered an unlocked position (Figure 3-6).

It is clearly evident that each joint possesses what is considered to be a normal physiologic range of motion. When is range of motion considered to be abnormal, or what we call *pathologic*? Pathologic range of motion can exist in one of two forms. First, if a joint movement is less than its normal active and/or passive physiological range of motion, it is considered to be pathological in nature. This deficit in available range of motion is commonly termed *hypomobile*. A hypomobile joint may exist from muscular weakness, neurological deficits, or internal derangement of structures such as bone or cartilage. Second, if a joint motion, actively or passively, exceeds what is considered to be the normal range of motion for that joint and for that individual, it is believed to be pathological. *Hypermobility* is typically a result of increased extensibility or instability of joint structures. While both a hypomobile and hypermobile joint may prevent ideal and functional range of motion at the respective joint, it is important not to forget that these conditions may also influence adjacent joints as outlined with respect to the kinematic chain principle.[9]

Arthrokinetics, on the other hand, is not only concerned with general movement but also with the causes behind movement itself. It is based on the foundation of Newton's second law of motion. Here, factors such as force, momentum, inertia, and resistance are considered in an attempt to determine why movement occurs and how changes in parameters may affect such movement. When applying these principles to rehabilitation, a clinician may be able to make small changes to apparatus or situations of an injured person that may ultimately lead to a more suitable setting for performance.

ACCESSORY RANGE OF MOTION

While joints move in physiologic motion that has been described in terms of angular motions, one must recognize that in order for this type of motion to achieve maximal ranges, a phenomena known as accessory range of motion must also occur. *Accessory range of motion* involves passive movement of joint surfaces that are measured in terms of millimeters.[15,16]

To understand how accessory motion works we must first examine the anatomy of the joint surfaces. Joint surfaces are classified as either *ovoid* or *sellar* in nature. An ovoid joint surface is one in which the relationship of two bones fit together as a result of one surface being concave and the other being convex (Figure 3-7). The degree to which the concave-convex relationship exists varies from one joint to another. In fact, some joint surfaces possess

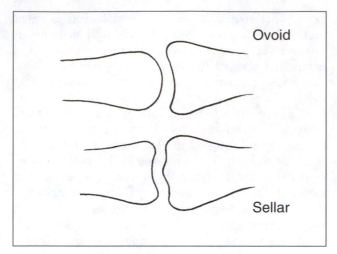

Figure 3-7. Ovoid and sellar joint relationships.

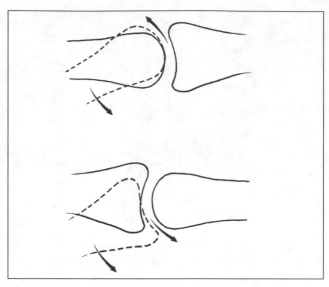

Figure 3-8. Convex-concave relationship of movement.

reciprocal relationships. That is, one bone has both a convex and a concave surface, as does the surface of the bone with which it articulates.[17] Therefore, depending on which direction plane movement occurs in, the surface area of a bone that is considered to be stationary or moving may be either convex or concave. This relationship is seen with sellar joints.

Since accessory movement is a passive activity, how then is movement accomplished? This is done by understanding what is called the *convex-concave rule of joint mobilization*. This rule states the following:

If the bone with the convexity is moved on the bone with the concavity, then the convex structure will move in the opposite direction to the bone segment (Figure 3-8).

If the bone with the concavity is moved on the bone with the convexity, the concave structure will move in the same direction as the bone segment (see Figure 3-8).

The concept of joint mobilization via accessory motion that follows the convex-concave rule is an extremely important component to rehabilitation of conditions with hypomobility as a result of adherent soft tissue structures. It is possible to apply normal physiologic (angular) stretching techniques to joints that are restricted of motion and not obtain positive results simply because it is the accessory (translatory) movements that are causing the restriction.

Mennell has termed this accessory motion *joint play*. He believes that a loss of joint play that is accompanied by pain is indicative of some type of joint dysfunction. Furthermore, he has outlined a process which he believes occurs during joint dysfunction:[16]

1. When a joint is not free to move, the muscles that move it cannot be free to move.
2. Muscles cannot be restored to normal if the joints that they move are not free to move.
3. Normal muscle function is dependent upon normal joint movement.
4. Impaired muscle function perpetuates and may cause deterioration in abnormal joints.

There are three types of accessory motion (Figure 3-9):

- *Rolling:* the multiple surface areas of a moving bone come in contact with multiple surface areas of a stationary bone.
- *Gliding or sliding:* the same surface area of a moving bone comes in contact with multiple surface areas of a stationary bone.
- *Spinning:* the multiple surface areas of a moving bone come in contact with the same surface area of a stationary bone.

Analogous to accessory motion within a joint is a car on an icy road. Initially, the car will drive down the road with multiple surface areas of a tire coming in contact with multiple surface areas of the road (rolling). When the car's brakes hit ice, the car skids. Here, the same surface area of the tire will come in contact with multiple surface areas of the road (gliding). The car will eventually come to a halt. When the driver then attempts to move the car again, the wheels may spin on the ice.

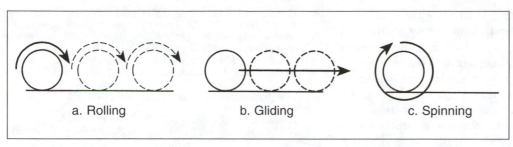

Figure 3-9. Types of accessory motion: a. rolling; b. gliding; c. spinning.

a. Rolling   b. Gliding   c. Spinning

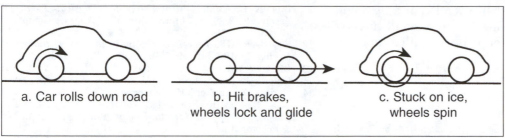

Figure 3-10. Accessory motion is analagous to a car and its tires: a. rolling; b. gliding; c. spinning.

a. Car rolls down road   b. Hit brakes, wheels lock and glide   c. Stuck on ice, wheels spin

Now, multiple surface areas of the tire will come in contact with the same surface area of the ice (spinning) (Figure 3-10).

We know that both rotary and translatory motion must exist in order to achieve maximal ranges of motion. We also know that each joint has a normative value with respect to this available motion. We must also be able to assess the quality of the end ranges of each of these movements. This is referred to as the joint's *end feel*. Numerous terms exist to describe the type of end feel that exists; however, some are more acceptable than others. In addition, some end feel terms have been classified as being both normal and abnormal, depending on the location and type of joint in which they are found to exist.[18]

A common end feel is labeled *bone-to-bone*. This is considered to be a normal end feel when one looks at extension of the elbow. Here, the olecranon process of the ulna and the olecranon fossa of the humerus come in complete contact with one another to form a closed pack position. This bone-to-bone contact limits further range of motion in the direction of elbow extension. However, if one were to feel a bone-to-bone end feel when moving into elbow flexion, this would not appear normal. Elbow flexion in most cases is limited by what is known as *soft tissue approximation*. The soft tissue components on the flexor side of the forearm come in contact with the soft tissue components on the anterior surface of the humerus, thus restricting any further elbow flexion from occurring.

A *capsular* end feel is also a normal end feel when found at the end ranges of external rotation of the shoulder, for example. However, if a person were limited in the direction of external rotation, a capsular end feel might still be found, indicating excessive capsular tightness. An *empty* end feel is often found and is indicative of no resistive structures that can be identified, but instead pain is usually the limiting factor preventing a person from further movement.

EFFECTS OF JOINT DEFORMATION

Because the movement of joints will create a change in the resting state of surrounding structures brought upon by the different types of forces described earlier, it is important to become familiar with the process of these structure's response to deformation.

When a structure fairly rapidly returns to its original state following deformation, it is said to be *elastic* in nature. This is seen most often with muscles and tendons surrounding a joint, whereby a musculotendinous junction will reach its elastic end range before quickly returning to its resting position. If, after deformation, a structure returns to its normal state but takes much more time doing so, it is said to have *crept* there. Structures that have visco-elastic properties, such as fibrocartilage, will typically follow this pattern. If a tissue does not return to its original state and remains deformed (typically elongated), it is said to have reached its *plastic* end range of motion.

At times with injury, tissue will neither return to its original state nor remain elongated or shortened. Instead, it will become *disrupted*. While disruption may occur to any joint structure, it takes on a different term depending on the structure that is involved. For instance, when a bone exceeds plastic end range, it will separate. This is referred to as a *fracture*. The same disruption that occurs to muscles, tendons, and ligaments is referred to as a *rupture*. More specifically, a rupture to a muscle or tendon is called a *strain*, whereas a rupture to a ligament is called a *sprain*. A plastic end range failure that involves either a tendon or a ligament as it proceeds to be connected to a small piece of bone, thus disrupting the bone, is called an *avulsion*.

References

1. Mulvihill ML. *Human Disease: A Systemic Approach*. 4th ed. Norwalk, Conn: Appleton & Lange; 1995.
2. Brooks GA, Fahey TD. *Exercise Physiology: Human Bioenergetics and its Applications*. New York, NY: Macmillan Publishing Company; 1985.
3. Osteoporosis. National Institutes of Health Consensus Development Conference Statement. 1984; 5(3).
4. Woo DL-Y. The effect of prolonged physical training on the properties of long bone: a study of Wolff's law. *J Bone Joint Surg Am*. 1981; 63-A:730.
5. Pratt NE. *Clinical Musculoskeletal Anatomy*. Philadelphia, Pa: JB Lippincott Company; 1991.
6. Hollinshead WH, Rosse C. *Textbook of Human Anatomy*. 4th ed. New York, NY: Harper & Row Publishers; 1985.
7. Moore KL, Agur AM. *Essential Clinical Anatomy*. Baltimore, Md: Williams & Wilkins; 1996.
8. Rasch PJ. *Kinesiology and Applied Anatomy*. 7th ed. Philadelphia, Pa: Lea & Febiger; 1989.
9. Norkin C, Levangie P. *Joint Structure and Function: A Comprehensive Analysis*. Philadelphia, Pa: FA Davis Company; 1983.
10. Lehmkuhl LD, Smith LK. *Brunnstrom's Clinical Kinesiology*. 4th ed. Philadelphia, Pa: FA Davis Company; 1983.
11. Lippert L. *Clinical Kinesiology for Physical Therapist Assistants*. 2nd ed. Philadelphia, Pa: FA Davis Company; 1994.
12. Soderberg GL. *Kinesiology: Application to Pathological Motion*. Baltimore, Md: Williams & Wilkins; 1986.
13. Brodal A. *Neurological Anatomy*. 3rd ed. New York, NY: Oxford University Press; 1981.
14. Nordin M, Frankel VH. Biomechanics of whole bones and bone tissue. In: Frankel VH, Nordin M (eds). *Basic Biomechanics of the Skeletal System*. Philadelphia, Pa: Lea & Febiger; 1980.
15. Maitland GD. *Peripheral Manipulation*. 2nd ed. Boston, Mass: Butterwoth; 1977.
16. Mennell JM. *Joint Pain: Diagnosis and Treatment Using Manipulative Techniques*. Boston, Mass: Little, Brown and Company; 1964.
17. MacConaill MA, Basmajian JV. *Muscles and Movements: A Basis for Human Kinesiology*. Baltimore, Md: Williams & Wilkins; 1969.
18. Wadsworth C. *Physical Examination of the Spine and Extremities*. Baltimore, Md: Williams and Wilkins; 1988.

1. List the four major types of tissue.

2. Describe the contents of bone and explain how certain physiological factors can influence the state of these structures.

3. Using a skeleton, identify long, flat, short, and irregular bones.

4. Explain the relationship between the stability and mobility of a joint.

5. What role does synovial fluid play within a joint capsule?

6. Review the classification of joints. Which joints are designed primarily for movement? What anatomical structures contribute to the movement of these joints and/or assist with joint stability?

7. What role do joint receptors play?

8. Using the spine as an example, demonstrate compression, tension, bending, torsion, and shear as each affects joint surfaces.

9. What is the key difference between *stress* and *strain* as they relate to joint forces?

10. Using the upper extremity as an example, demonstrate the difference between an open and closed kinematic activity.

11. Define arthrokinematics and arthokinetics. How do these differ?

12. Explain the importance of accessory motion. List the major types of accessory motion and give an example of each within the body.

13. Demonstrate the convex-concave rule using an anatomical model.

14. Name the different types of capsular end feels. Identify both normal and abnormal end feels using specific joints of the body.

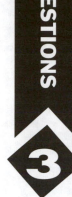

CHAPTER 4

MUSCLE STRUCTURE AND FUNCTION

Jeff G. Konin, MEd, ATC, MPT

OBJECTIVES

After completion of this chapter, the reader will be able to:

DIDACTIC

1. Identify the various ways that muscles can be classified.
2. Describe different muscle fiber arrangements and give an example of each.
3. Define properties of a muscle to include contractibility, irritability, extensibility, and elasticity.
4. Explain the roles of muscles as they relate to mobility and stability.
5. Describe the length-tension relationship of a muscle and explain its relevance to movement.
6. Differentiate between active and passive insufficiency.
7. Differentiate between isometric, isotonic, and isokinetic muscle contractions.

PRACTICAL

1. Observe the contraction of muscles, including those that are parallel and oblique in nature.
2. Identify muscles in the resting state versus a contractile state.
3. Recognize fiber characteristics of muscles based on daily physical stresses.
4. Identify a joint movement and determine those muscles that are prime movers, synergists, and antagonists.
5. Demonstrate passive and active insufficiency as it relates to two-joint muscles.
6. Perform isometric, isotonic, and isokinetic exercises and demonstrate the differences between each.
7. Demonstrate and utilize those muscles capable of performing functionally in reverse actions.

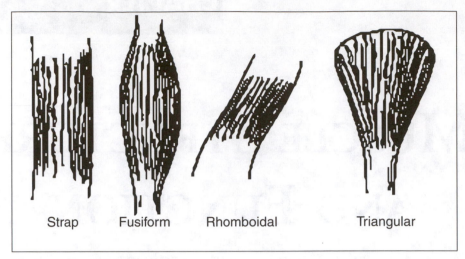

Figure 4-1. Parallel muscle fibers.

MUSCLE STRUCTURE

The function of skeletal muscle is similar to the function of joint structures in that it is designed to meet the body's need for functional mobility and stability. Muscles are classified as *active* or *noninert tissue*. That is, they have the potential to contract and create movement as a result of that contraction. The make-up of the actual tissue itself is portrayed in many ways and forms within the body. However, one commonality of all muscle tissue is their basic type of attachment. A muscle can be found attached on one end to a bone, while the other end is attached to a tendon that will then connect the muscle to a bone. This area where the tendon actually connects the muscle to the bone is referred to as the *musculotendinous junction*. Muscles are further classified in many ways. These include the type of muscle fiber arrangement, the location of the muscle, the action of the muscle, and the number of heads that a muscle contains, among others.

Muscle Fiber Arrangement

In general, two types of arrangements of muscle fiber exist: *parallel* and *oblique*. Parallel muscle fibers tend to be longer in length, thus allowing for a greater potential range of motion. By contrast, oblique fibers tend to be shorter in length. However, oblique arrangements may contain more fibers per a given area of muscle tissue.[1-3]

Parallel muscle fibers can be broken down into four sub-categories (Figure 4-1):

1. **Strap:** long and thin with fibers running the entire length of the muscle (eg, sartorius).

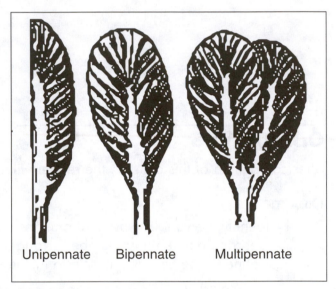

Figure 4-2. Oblique muscle fibers.

2. **Fusiform:** spindle-shaped, whereby they are wider in the middle and taper off at both ends (eg, brachialis).
3. **Rhomboid:** a flat muscle, rectangular or square-like (eg, rhomboids, pronator quadratus).
4. **Triangular:** flat and fan-shaped, with fibers coming from a narrow attachment at one end and a broad attachment on the other (eg, pectoralis major).

Oblique muscle fibers can be broken down into three sub-categories (Figure 4-2):

1. **Unipennate:** a series of short fibers attached diagonally along the length of a central tendon and appear like a one-sided feather (eg, tibialis posterior of ankle).

Table 4-1
Skeletal Muscle Fiber Characteristics

	FG	FOG	SO
Muscle color	white	red	red
Muscle diameter	large	medium	small
Myoglobin content	low	medium	high
Contractile speed	fast	fast	slow
Fatigue rate	fast	medium	slow
Size of motor unit	large	medium	small
Conduction velocity	fast	fast	slow

2. **Bipennate:** fibers that are obliquely attached to both sides of a central tendon and look like a feather (eg, rectus femoris).
3. **Multipennate:** many tendons with oblique fibers (eg, deltoid, subscapularis).

Properties of Muscle Structure

A muscle has been described as a contractile tissue. This property, along with some others, distinguish muscle tissue from all others within the body. *Contractibility* describes the process of a muscle shortening when it actively contracts. During this process, it possesses the ability to develop tension against a resistance. Typically, muscles will respond by contracting when a stimulus is activated. The stimulus can be a motor nerve within the body or it can be from an externally induced electrical charge, such as seen during rehabilitation of injuries using electrical therapeutic modalities. A stimulus can also be chemical or mechanical in nature. This ability of a muscle to respond to a stimulus is called *irritability*.[1]

When a muscle is contracted and shortened, ultimately it should return to its original position or state. This is called the *resting state*. Lengthening of a muscle occurs not only following its shortening, but also when a force is applied that will subsequently increase the length of a muscle. The ability of a muscle to lengthen to its resting state, or stretch beyond this state, is referred to as a muscle's *extensibility*. A muscle that has the capability of shortening or lengthening and then returning to its normal state once a force or contraction is removed is said to be *elastic*. A rubber band is an example of a structure that is elastic. Gum, on the other hand, is extensible, but not elastic.

Muscle Fiber Types

A muscle's fiber type helps to determine the actual characteristics of a muscle with respect to its function. Muscles have been described as being 1. fast-twitch glycolytic (FG); 2. fast-twitch oxidative/glycolytic (FOG); and 3. slow-twitch oxidative (SO).[4-6] Each of these types of skeletal muscle fibers possess varying amounts of oxygen and glycogen. Those fibers that contain higher percentages of oxygen are primarily designed for long duration, endurance type activities. By contrast, the fibers containing higher percentages of glycogen are designed for short-term power type activities. The fast-twitch oxidative/glycolytic fibers contain a fairly equal percentage of both components but have the ability to adapt to becoming more favorable to one versus the other through training methods that facilitate the use and need for a certain type (Table 4-1).

THE ROLE OF MUSCLES

As muscles come in different shapes, sizes, and structural components, they also serve many roles. Globally, muscles are designed to initiate and assist with joint movement as well as to help control and resist joint movement by stabilizing bony articulations. To better understand the role that muscles play, we need to label muscles with respect to the type of function they serve.

Any muscle that contracts and creates joint movement is considered to be a *mover* or *agonist*. Muscles can be movers of single joints in a single direction, such as the soleus with plantarflexion. Muscles can also be movers of more than one joint. This is seen with the rectus femoris, as it can create knee extension as well as hip flexion.

As discussed earlier, the type, size, and location of a muscle all play a role in determining the overall ability of a muscle to create movement. Muscles that play major roles in causing movement about a certain joint are classified as being *prime movers*. For example, the deltoid muscle is a prime mover of the glenohumeral joint. Other muscles may assist with actual joint movements but do not necessarily contribute to the motion with such a large degree of force. These muscles are referred to as *assistive movers*. The soleus is a good example of an assistive mover, as it assists the larger gastrocnemius to plantarflex the foot. Many times, more than one prime mover or assistive mover may exist during a joint motion. It is not always definitive as to whether a muscle is a primary or secondary mover at a joint.

The contraction of a muscle that leads to joint motion in a particular direction must be limited by opposing forces. In Chapter 3, we discussed various types of end feels that are found to identify the end range of motion in a single direction. Muscles serve not only to move joints, but also to resist movement. When a muscle contracts and causes the movement of a joint in the direction opposite to that previously caused by another muscle, this former muscle is said to be an *antagonist*. Examination of the knee joint exemplifies a relationship between an agonist and antagonist muscle group. During knee extension, the quadriceps contract to extend the knee, serving as the prime movers, while contraction and shortening of the hamstrings serve to oppose this movement, a function of an antagonistic muscle group. During knee flexion, the hamstring muscle group would be considered the agonist and the quadriceps group the antagonist.

Muscles can also serve as *synergists*. A synergistic muscle is one that assists an agonistic muscle with a movement by either contracting to help create the movement or by helping to stabilize a structure, thus preventing an unwanted movement. At the wrist, muscles such as the extensor carpi ulnaris and the extensor carpi radialis longus and brevis are all agonists to wrist extension. The extensor digitorum communis, by way of its origin and insertion also crossing the wrist, serves as a synergist to help extend the wrist.

One would expect a muscle to contract and shorten from both ends, thus evenly shortening toward its central location. This should be a normal response of a muscle. However, there are times when this occurs and ideal movement is not achieved. This is due to the inability of one end of the muscle to become fixated. To prevent this, some muscles serve as stabilizers or fixators in an attempt to fixate one end of a muscle. A stabilizing muscle anchors or supports a bone so that another muscle can perform efficiently.[7] This is seen in many instances throughout the body, perhaps none more common than when one throws an object. Here, if a person's arm reached forward when releasing the object, you would expect the scapulae to follow in suit. However, muscles such as the rhomboids act to stabilize the scapula and allow for more efficient use of the rotator cuff muscles.

As muscles help to mobilize and stabilize joints, it is largely believed that the proximity of a muscle's proximal and distal attachments to the joint that is being acted upon determine, to a certain extent, the role of the muscle. Based on this proximity, muscles are referred to as either spurt or shunt.[7-9] A *spurt* muscle has its proximal attachments further away from the joint that is being acted upon, while its distal attachment is closer to the joint. This typically creates a large rotary component to movement, allowing for motion to occur. *Shunt* muscles possess a proximal attachment closer to the joint of action and a distal attachment further away. In this situation, a muscle tends to pull bones together, creating a more translatory effect and acting as a stabilizer to joint motion. Some muscles cross two joints and are likely to possess spurt characteristics at one joint and shunt characteristics at the other.

LENGTH-TENSION RELATIONSHIP OF MUSCLES

Muscles not only serve to move joints, but they do this in a manner whereby tension is developed that is used to exert a force. *Tension* is the actual magnitude of force that is developed. Typically, the elongating of a muscle will act to build this tension while the tension is relieved when the muscle returns to its original state or length.

Tension can be developed through active or passive measures. *Active tension* is brought upon by the contractile elements that lie within the muscle itself. This occurs through a muscle contraction or shortening. The potential to develop active tension depends on a number of factors[8] (Table 4-2). *Passive tension*, on the other hand, is developed by a change of position in the passive elastic components. With passive tension, no muscle contraction is needed.[10-11]

Table 4-2
Factors Related to Producing Active Tension

- ✔ Frequency of motor units firing
- ✔ Number of motor units firing
- ✔ Size of motor units firing
- ✔ Type of motor units firing
- ✔ Number of muscle fibers in a cross-section of the muscle

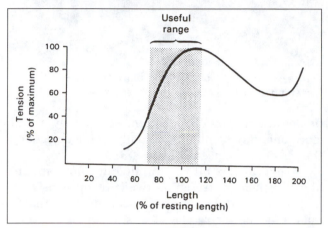

Figure 4-3. Length-tension relationship of a muscle (reprinted with permission from Lehmkuhl LD, Smith LK. *Brunnstrom's Clinical Kinesiology.* 4th ed. Philadelphia, Pa: FA Davis; 1983).

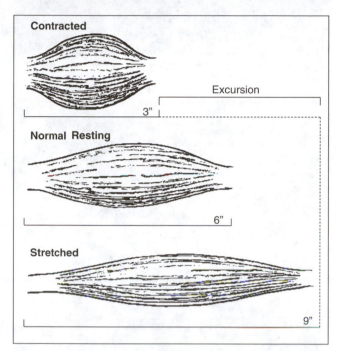

Figure 4-4. Excursion of a muscle.

There is a direct relationship between the length of a muscle and the tension it is capable of generating. The position in which a muscle is able to generate maximal tension is called the optimal length.[12] This position is considered to be close to the muscle's resting position, at 10% beyond the length of the resting length[11] (Figure 4-3). It is important to remember that a muscle that is connected on both ends may not be at its true resting length, since this might actually occur with the muscle needing to be slightly more elongated. When attached, it is unable to reach these lengths.

The length that a muscle is measured by when it shortens and expands is known as the *excursion* of a muscle. It is believed that a muscle can shorten to about one-half of its normal resting length and elongate to about twice as far as it can be shortened[1] (Figure 4-4).

PASSIVE AND ACTIVE INSUFFICIENCY

When muscles become elongated over two joints simultaneously, they may reach a state of *passive insufficiency*.[1,8,10] When this occurs, further motion of the muscle will be limited as a result. To better understand this concept, one can look at how hamstring flexibility is altered when the muscle is maximally stretched over one versus two joints. When one flexes the hip with the knees in flexion, the hamstrings are only maximally stretched over the hip joint and loose behind the knee joint. Here, about 115° to 125° of hip flexion may be accomplished. Simply extending the knee with the hips flexed now places the hamstrings in a taut position at both joints. When this occurs, the amount of excursion for hip flexion will be limited (Figures 4-5a and 4-5b).

This concept can be applied to normal movement as well as pathologic movement. Conditions such as muscle tightness, muscle spasticity, and adhesions may predispose one to having passively insufficient muscles. However, this is not always a deterring situation.[13]

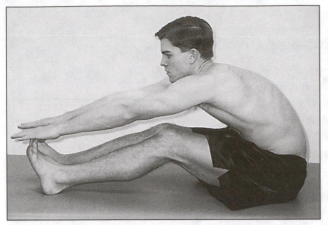

Figure 4-5a. Example of hamstring muscles as they cross the knee.

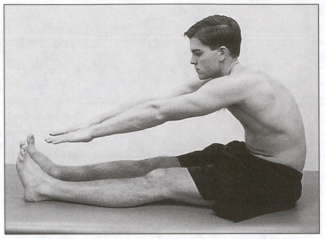

Figure 4-5b. Example of passive insufficiency in which the hamstring muscles are taut at the hip and knee.

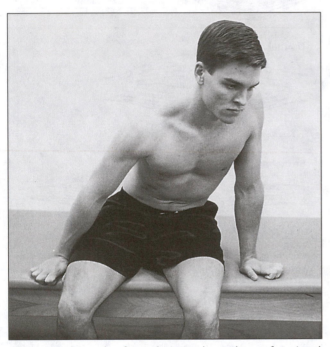

Figure 4-6. Example of tenodesis used to enhance functional performance.

The passive tension that is created by two-joint muscles can actually produce a functional movement of a joint. This process is called *tenodesis* and can be performed when a two-joint muscle is stretched over both joints. The most common practical example of this occurs at the wrist. With the wrist in flexion, one can achieve full extension of the fingers. However, when the wrist is put into extension, the fingers naturally begin to flex, and extension of the fingers is much harder to obtain. This principle is often used with spinal cord injured patients who may have use of the wrist extensors but not the wrist and finger flexors. In this case, actively extending the wrist will assist in flexing the fingers. This becomes extremely useful since one may be able to actually grasp objects by the tension produced (Figure 4-6).

From a flexibility standpoint, one should always consider stretching two-joint muscles with both ends taut. This way you can be sure that a muscle is being stretched to its maximal position. When stretching with the muscle slack across one joint, you cannot always be sure if the stretch that is being performed is utilizing the maximal excursion of the muscle.

The concept of *active insufficiency* differs from that of passive insufficiency in that it relates to a force production measurement as opposed to range of motion excursion. Remember that all joints have an optimal length-tension relationship. When a muscle is shortened, it is not capable of producing optimal tension or force. Since we have the ability to influence the position of two-joint muscles, this concept can be seen quite evidently. For example, we can look at the wrist flexor muscle group to highlight this principle.

If you were to measure the grip strength of an individual, you would see that the force produced by the finger flexors is much greater, while the wrist is in a position of extension versus flexion. In fact, the position of greatest force production relative to grip strength occurs when the wrist is in slight extension. This occurs as a result of the length changes of the flexor tendons while the wrist is moved from flexion to extension.

This concept, while used in rehabilitation quite frequently, is also used during the teaching of self-defense classes. When a person is fighting off an attacker, he or she is told to try to grab the attacker's wrist and maximally flex it in an effort to

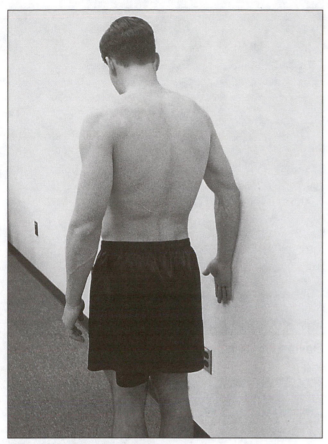

Figure 4-7. Isometric exercise.

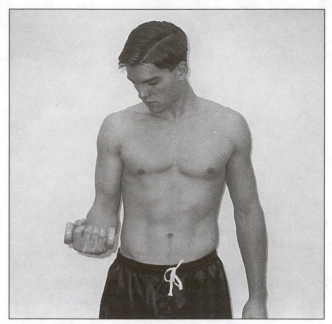

Figure 4-8. Isotonic exercise.

reduce the ability of the attacker to produce force through the hands.

TYPES OF MUSCLE CONTRACTIONS

Three basic, but essential, types of muscular contractions occur within the body. These are *isometric, isotonic,* and *isokinetic*. All three types can occur in each individual muscle, and each type plays an important role within a given function. Again, the contraction of a muscle will relate to the mobility or stability of a joint.

It is possible for a muscle to develop tension against a given resistance without actually shortening or lengthening in a way that will produce excursion. This is referred to as an isometric contraction. This occurs when the tension of the muscle is insufficient against the resistive force, therefore not changing the angle at the given joint. The term isometric comes from the Greek word "isos," meaning equal, and the term "metron," meaning measure.[10] Isometric exercises are used as a form of rehabilitation when one wants to strengthen the muscles around a joint without producing any joint movement or deformation. (Figure 4-7).

Isotonic contractions occur when a muscle is able to overcome a resistive force and in turn produce a movement of a particular joint angle. The term "tonus" also comes from Greek origin and refers to tension.[10] Technically, one would infer this to mean that the muscle remains in equal tension throughout its contraction. However, this can be somewhat confusing. With isotonic forms of exercise, the resistance (or weight) remains the same throughout the exercise. Therefore, the muscle actually changes its tension in an effort to move the weight throughout the various ranges of joint motion (Figure 4-8).

Isotonic contractions are actually classified in terms of whether they shorten a muscle or lengthen it. Contractions that are performed in which the result is muscle shortening is termed *concentric*. A concentric muscle contraction can be seen when a person lifts a dumbbell weight toward his or her chest with the help of the biceps muscle. Upon returning the weight to the original joint position, the muscle will undergo a lengthening process. During this time, it is still contracting and assisting to move the resistance throughout a joint range. When the muscle lengthens in this fashion, it is said to be contracting in an *eccentric* manner (Figures 4-9a and 4-9b).

The third type of muscle contraction is isokinetic. The term "kinetos" is also a Greek word meaning moving or movement. So an isokinetic

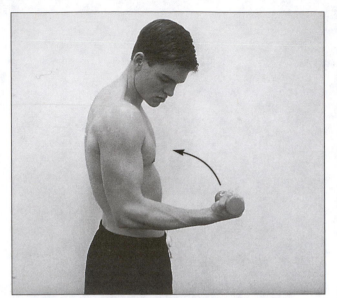

Figure 4-9a. Concentric exercise of the biceps muscle.

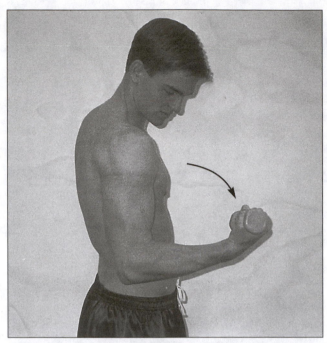

Figure 4-9b. Eccentric exercise of the biceps muscle.

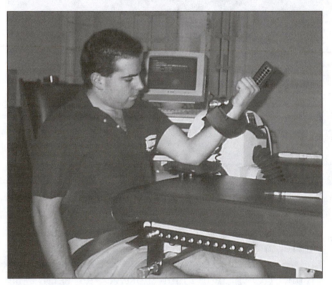

Figure 4-10. Example of an isokinetic machine.

contraction is one in which the muscle creates the same or equal rate or speed of movement throughout joint angle changes. The main characteristic of an isokinetic contraction is that the resistance of the weight or object is able to accommodate to the position that the muscle is in at a given joint angle. This allows for the ability to put out a maximal contraction utilizing the length-tension relationship principles throughout the entire range of motion.[14] Since a muscle is not as capable of producing as much tension at the beginning or end ranges of motion as it is in its optimal lengthened position, a person will have difficulty moving a weight during a knee extension exercise in these ranges as opposed to when the joint is midway through its range of motion. However, during an isokinetic contraction, the weight is able to adjust to the tension and angle of the joint so that the resistance feels the same regardless of the joint angle during contraction. This is accomplished through specially designed machines and devices (Figure 4-10).

A nice feature of exercising in an isokinetic mode is that the accommodating resistance responds to the amount of tension that a person develops. For instance, the greater tension that is produced with a muscle contraction, the harder the machine will resist that action. Likewise, when one decreases the effort, the resistance lessens. This is an important concept built into isokinetic dynamometers that serves as a safety feature. If a person develops pain during a bout of exercise, he or she can simply stop exerting force and the machine will instantaneously cut off its resistance. This is unable to be accomplished during isotonic contractions, as the resistance will remain the same even when a person halts an effort, thus having the potential for injury.

REVERSE MUSCLE ACTION

To this point, we have discussed the normal directional movement of a muscle contraction. That is, in most cases when a muscle contracts, the

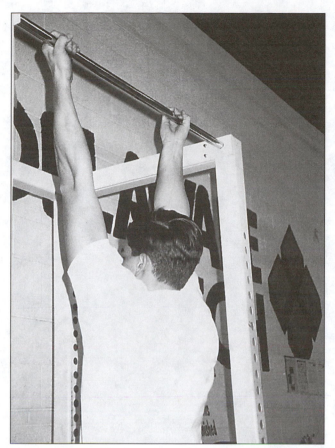 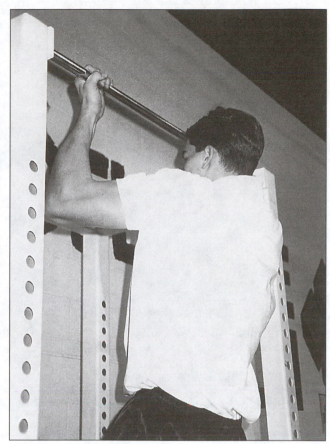

Figure 4-11 a and b. Reverse muscle action of the biceps during a pull-up.

proximal attachment or origin serves as a stabilizing component, while the distal attachment or insertion becomes the moving component. Because this does not always occur within the human body, the terms *proximal attachment* and *distal attachment* are more appropriate to use, as opposed to origin and insertion.

Consider the previous example of a person performing an elbow flexion exercise using the biceps brachii against resistance. In this case, the biceps long head proximal attachment at the supraglenoid tubercle remains stable while the contraction of the muscle pulls on the distal attachment at the radial tuberosity. This is the normal directional action of joint movement and will typically occur when the distal attachment is an open kinetic chain.

Now look at what happens when a person does a pull-up. Here, the same biceps brachii muscle is contracting to perform elbow flexion. However, in the closed kinetic chain, the distal attachment is now fixed on the bar, and the proximal attachment moves as the joint angle decreases. This type of muscle contraction that changes the joint angle is referred to as *reverse action* (Figures 4-11 a and b).

References

1. Lippert L. *Clinical Kinesiology for Physical Therapist Assistants*. 2nd ed. Philadelphia, Pa: FA Davis Company; 1994.
2. Moore K. *Clinically Oriented Anatomy*. 2nd ed. Baltimore, Md: Williams & Wilkins; 1985.
3. Pratt NE. *Clinical Musculoskeletal Anatomy*. Philadelphia, Pa: JB Lippincott Company; 1991.
4. Brooks GA, Fahey TD. *Exercise Physiology: Human Bioenergettics and its Applications*. New York, NY: Macmillan Publishing Company; 1985.
5. McArdle WD, Katch FI, Katch VL. *Exercise Physiology: Energy, Nutrition and Human Performance*. 3rd ed. Philadelphia, Pa: Lea & Febiger; 1991.
6. Karlsson J, Jacobs I. Onset of blood lactate accumulation during muscular exercise as a threshold concept: Part 1. Theoretical considerations. *Int J Sports Med*. 1982; 3:190.
7. Rasch PJ. *Kinesiology and Applied Anatomy*. 7th ed. Philadelphia, Pa: Lea & Febiger; 1989.
8. Norkin C, Levangie P. *Joint Structure and Function: A Comprehensive Analysis*. Philadelphia, Pa: FA Davis Company; 1983.
9. Soderberg GL. *Kinesiology: Application to Pathological Motion*. Baltimore, Md: Williams & Wilkins; 1986.
10. Lehmkuhl LD, Smith LK. *Brunnstrom's Clinical Kinesiology*. 4th ed. Philadelphia, Pa: FA Davis Company; 1983.
11. Ramsey RW, Street SF. Isometric length-tension diagram of isolated skeletal muscle fibers of a frog. *Journal of Cellular and Comparative Physiology*. 1940; 15:11.

12. Gowitzke BA, Milner M. *Understanding the Scientific Basis for Human Movement.* 2nd ed. Baltimore, Md: Williams & Wilkins; 1980.

13. Guyton AC. *Basic Neuroscience.* 2nd ed. Philadelphia, Pa: WB Saunders Company; 1991.

14. Hislop HJ, Perrine JJ. The isokinetic concept of exercise. *Phys Ther.* 1967; 47:114.

1. Explain the difference between parallel and oblique muscle fibers and give an example of each subtype.

2. What are the different muscle fiber types in the body that relate to oxidative function?

3. Define contractibility, irritability, extensibility, and elasticity.

4. How is a muscle affected by its length-tension relationship?

5. Using the hamstring muscle group, demonstrate how you would perform each of the following exercises: isometric, isotonic, and isokinetic.

6. How do concentric and eccentric exercises differ from one another? Do these types of contractions have any similarities or differences when compared to reverse muscle action contractions?

7. Using the quadriceps muscle group, demonstrate both active and passive insufficiency. What is the major difference between these two concepts?

8. How is tenodesis accomplished at the wrist? Can this be performed at other joints in the body?

9. Using the elbow joint as an example, which muscle surfaces serve as agonists versus antagonists during elbow flexion and extension?

STUDY QUESTIONS 4

CHAPTER 5

PRINCIPLES OF TISSUE REPAIR

Jeff G. Konin, MEd, ATC, MPT

OBJECTIVES

After completion of this chapter, the reader will be able to:

DIDACTIC

1. Identify the three main phases of tissue healing and describe the major events of each phase.
2. Identify the five main signs/symptoms associated with inflammation.
3. Compare healing properties of different tissue types.
4. Recognize internal and external factors that may affect tissue healing.
5. Explain how mobilization plays an important role in tissue healing.

PRACTICAL

1. Identify a given injury and explain how the phases of tissue healing affect the involved tissue.
2. Look for characteristic signs/symptoms of an injury and recognize these as being a normal process of inflammation.
3. Demonstrate mobilization techniques to various tissues and examine normal movement.
4. Predict how movement will be affected following an injury that results in inflammation and subsequent tissue healing and repair.

INTRODUCTION

When one studies the principles of kinesiology, it is important to consider the actual properties of each tissue independently. Any disturbance in a single tissue that is part of a bodily movement can alter the outcome of the desired movement. Structures that are hyper- or hypomobile not only affect the overall movement, but need to be addressed and considered during the recovery process of the particular tissue involved. The purpose of this chapter is to outline the phases of healing as they reflect specific tissue components. Furthermore, the importance of how this affects clinical applications will be discussed with respect to human movement. For a more indepth look at the physiology and biochemistry of individual tissues, refer to the list of suggested readings at the end of the chapter.

TISSUE HEALING

Understanding the make-up of normal tissue is not sufficient enough for a clinician to deal with human movement. Movement in itself is influenced by many factors. One of these factors is an alteration of the make-up as a result of injury or impairment. When this occurs, the respective tissue undergoes a series of events in an attempt to return to its pre-morbid functioning state. While much information is published on the topic of tissue repair and wound healing, the process has yet to be entirely understood.[1] However, it is essential that a clinician working with a subject who is being treated for movement dysfunction understand to the best of his or her ability how the principles of healing will affect a person's return to activities of daily living.

Just as soon as a tissue becomes insulted, the process of healing begins. This process has been described by many authors using various terminology. Essentially, the healing process takes place in three phases: *inflammation*, *repair*, and *remodeling*.[2-11] It is important to understand, however, that each of these phases lacks a finite and clear beginning and end, and that they in fact overlap each other in most, if not all, instances (Figure 5-1).

Inflammation Phase

This first phase is the body's initial response to injury. The inflammation phase serves as a protective mechanism as well as the initiation of healing.

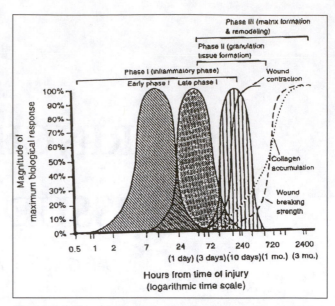

Figure 5-1. Phases of tissue healing (reprinted with permission from Kloth LC, McCulloh JM, Feedar JA, eds. *Wound Healing Alternatives in Management*. Philadelphia, Pa: FA Davis; 1990).

The main purpose of the inflammatory reaction is to remove all foreign debris, thereby reducing the likelihood of infection so that optimal wound healing can occur.[12] During this phase, a series of biochemical, vascular, and cellular events occur to facilitate tissue repair. While most believe that the inflammation phase lasts up to 4 days, others believe it can last up to 5 days and longer.[2,4-7,9,11,13-18]

The inflammation phase is characterized by an immediate vasoconstriction lasting for a few minutes, which is soon followed by vasodilation, resulting in an increased flow of circulation to the involved area. Cellular permeability increases, allowing for fluids such as blood and plasma to enter the area. Platelets from the blood bind to collagen, thus releasing phospholipids that will aid in stimulating a clotting mechanism. In addition, fibrin also enters the area to eventually form the wound's only source of tensile strength during this phase.[9]

Within hours, polymorphonuclear leukocytes (PMNs) and mast cells migrate to the area to help fight off foreign bodies that attempt to invade the wound. Mast cells contain heparin (an anti-coagulant) and histamine. Neutrophils, a type of leukocyte, play a role in phagocytosis. That is, they ingest small debris such as bacteria and dead cells to fight against infection and/or further injury. Over the first few days, monocytic cells assist the PMNs in debriding the area of necrotic tissue and foreign bacteria. Once cleansed, fibroblasts travel to the area and begin the process of collagen lay-down that will eventually form scar tissue.[2] Chemically, histamine, serotonin, and bradykinin are released and travel to the injured area. Histamine is a major vasodilator, serotonin a vaso-constrictor, and bradykinin serves to increase cel-lular permeability, thus potentially increasing one's perception of pain.[19]

CLINICAL IMPLICATIONS

During the inflammation phase, a person will experience a number of cardinal signs/symptoms. These include swelling (tumor), redness (rubor), heat (calor), pain (dolor), and loss of function (func-tio laesa).[11,17,18,20,21] Loss of function has been reported to be a result of a combination of two bod-ily alterations. First, it is believed that there is a neurological reflex-inhibiting movement secondary to pain. Realistically, this tells a person that when an injured structure is moved, it will hurt. In addi-tion, there may be enough edema present that it can, in and of itself, restrict complete and normal joint range of motion.[18,22] Furthermore, pressure and/or chemical irritation of pain-producing free nerve endings may also elicit a feeling of discom-fort.[12] Any tissue damage, especially that of a mus-culotendinous type, can result in a deficit of force production.[23] While a keen clinician should always concentrate on identifying and addressing the cause of tissue damage, it is critically important to address these cardinal symptoms of the inflamma-tion phase in an attempt to maintain and return one to optimal function as safely and quickly as possible. The presence of persistent irritants can not only lead to a loss of function, but can adverse-ly affect wound healing and result in a much more difficult time counteracting infection.[8,12]

Repair Phase

The commencement of the repair phase is char-acterized by an accumulation of fibroplasts, myofi-broblasts, and endothelial cells.[2,4,7,9,16-18,24-27] These cells combine with the capillary system to form granulation tissue. This process of new cell creation occurs simultaneously with cell destruc-tion and the removal of debris from the area. Success of this phase depends upon elimination of debris and the regeneration of epithelial cells and production of fibroplasts.[20] Within hours of the ini-tial tissue damage, the re-epithelialization process of superficial skin wounds is initiated.[28-29] As a result of not having fully mature granulation, the fibers of the structure are thin and weak in nature,

and the tensile strength of the area may be at its lowest level during this time.[5,8,18] Not only is the collagenous formation of the tissue vulnerable to breakdown, the vascular system is also weak at this phase and is sensitive to bleeding.

It is believed that between the period of 7 and 10 days, the amount of localized collagen increases significantly, thus increasing the overall strength of the tissue.[9,13,18,26] This occurs for about 2 to 3 weeks, at which point the tissue loses some fluid and the collagen fibers become even more mature and densely packed together.[4,5,9]

CLINICAL IMPLICATIONS

Collagen has no consistent organization to it during the early phases, and the type of scar that appears is red and swollen, easily damaged, and remains tender to stretch or pressure.[1] Although range of motion provides the ideal stimulus for col-lagen regeneration, repeated trauma to the wound surface through excessive skin stretching during this phase may interfere with healing.[20,30] It is the experience of the clinician that must be utilized to determine the exact amount of movement that an injured tissue can tolerate without undergoing fur-ther damage during the repair phase.

When working with healing tissue during the repair phase, it is important to remember that the facilitation of circulation, especially through move-ment, may be beneficial in eliminating debris from the area. Even though during this phase tissue remains somewhat sensitive to stretch, it now begins to strengthen itself. Therefore, careful con-trolled movement is most beneficial at this time of healing.

Remodeling Phase

The third phase of tissue healing is referred to as the remodeling phase. The ultimate goal of the remodeling phase is to restore tissue function to as close to normal as possible.[12] Again, there is a gen-eral overlapping of all the phases, though it is believed that the remodeling phase takes place pre-dominantly from weeks 3 to 6. During this time, an increase in both the production of scar tissue and the strength of its fibers are seen.[20-31] Depending on the type of tissue involved, this process can actually last anywhere from 3 months to 2 years.[2,4,9,11,26,32-36] During this time, the healing tissue takes on more of a fibrous personality as opposed to a cellular make-up.[37] By the end of the sixth week, the vascu-larity of the scar matches that of the skin lying adja-cent, and the sensitivity of the area is reduced.[1,38]

One note of importance is that the tensile strength of newly formed collagen is correlated to the mechanical forces that are imposed on the tissue during this phase. More specifically, forces applied to a ligament, for example, will develop strength specifically in the direction that the force is applied[39-40] (Figure 5-2). Initially following the injury to the tissue, little tensile strength is lost. However, within days, a respective amount of tensile strength can be lost.[13,14,16,41-42] Like the repair phase, if too early or too much force is placed on the tissue, the results could be adverse.[34,43-44]

CLINICAL IMPLICATIONS

A clinician must know when it is appropriate to mobilize a healing muscle, tendon, ligament, or any other structure so as not to create further damage. More so, the actual amount of force that can be administered to each healing tissue must be understood. Under practical situations, these decisions may not appear as black and white to the novice clinician. However, if too much force is placed on a healing tissue or if aggressive mobilization is performed too early, further delays in the healing process can occur. Likewise, prolonged immobilization may consequently lead to weaker tissue formation and/or deficits in range of motion via unwanted collagen laydown.

Since the time frame of healing during the remodeling phase can last up to 2 years, it is important to continue to promote optimal healing in any tissue that has undergone an inflammatory response. Unfortunately, a typical scenario consists of a person decreasing the type of care and attention given to an injury once the intolerable pain has subsided. It is the responsibility of the practicing clinician to explain the importance of prolonged rehabilitation of a patient so that maximum benefit is achieved throughout the entire healing process.

SPECIFIC TISSUE HEALING PROPERTIES

Muscle

For the most part, muscle tissue cells are permanent and have little to no capacity for regeneration. However, there are reserve cells that exist within the membrane of a muscle fiber that contribute to the formation of new skeletal muscle.[15] Following damage to muscle cells, scar tissue will

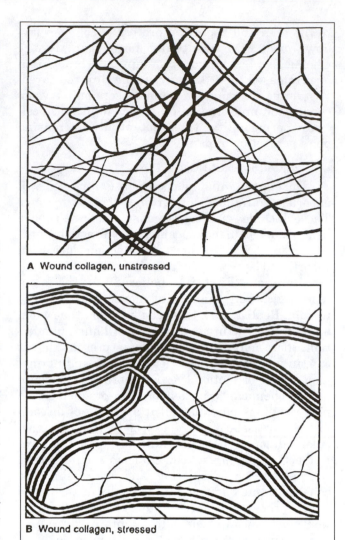

Figure 5-2. A. Unstressed and B. stressed wound collagen. In the wound subjected to stress, collagen reorganizes with larger, more parallel alligned fibers (reprinted with permission from Hertling D, Kessler RM. *Management of Common Musculoskeletal Disorders: Physical Therapy Principles and Methods.* Philadelphia, Pa: JB Lippincott; 1996).

typically develop, and the muscle unit will potentially lose a good portion of its tensile strength. However, muscle tissue may reach its near normal tensile strength level in 7 to 11 days.[14-15] This process of regaining tensile strength is dependent upon the maturity of the replaced collagen fibers as is described by the principles of *Wolff's law*.[44] Wolff's law simply states that a bone will respond to the amount of physical stresses that it undergoes.

Pain is a common symptom associated with muscle injury and has been reported to present itself in one of three ways:

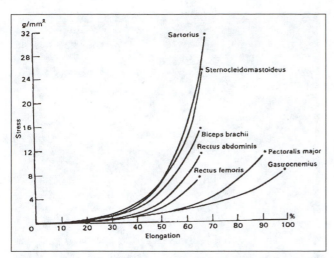

Figure 5-3. Stress-strain plots derived from the application of tension to skeletal muscle in 29-year-olds (reprinted from Yamada H. In: Evans FG, ed. *Strength of Biological Materials.* Baltimore, Md: Williams & Wilkins; 1970).

- Delayed onset muscle soreness
- Acute muscle soreness
- Injury-related soreness[45]

Delayed onset muscle soreness (DOMS) usually exists between 1 to 2 days post-injury. It is accompanied by palpable tenderness, a feeling of muscle stiffness, and a possible loss of range of motion. DOMS is believed to be a result of reduced blood flow and oxygen to the injured tissue.[46]

Acute muscle soreness occurs during or very shortly after a bout of exercise. It is also believed to be caused by a lack of oxygen to the muscular tissue, seen especially with isometric contractions.[45] Acute muscle soreness is often reported as a burning sensation that is commonly seen with weight-lifting activities.

Injury-related muscle soreness is actual tissue damage that is encountered as a result of an imbalance between the agonist and antagonist muscle groups of the respected tissue. Often, this is seen with rapid joint movements, thus placing a large strain on the muscular tissue. Different muscles within the body are able to accommodate varying levels of stress and strain[47] (Figure 5-3).

A muscle that is acting without the capability of utilizing all of its fibers will be at a disadvantage with respect to force production. This may alter a clinician's thought process when determining the amount of resistance and type of contraction that is desired to be performed during rehabilitation. In addition, it is possible to have altered length-tension relationships as a result of an injury that could also change force production. These factors must be considered when designing rehabilitation programs since pre-morbid levels of function may not be reached early in the programs, if at all.

Tendon

Injury to a tendon may include anything from a partial tearing to a complete rupture. Inflammation and vascular insult will usually accompany tendon damage. Because collagen fibers are arranged in a parallel form, tendons can typically tolerate high tensile loads.[47] Nordin and Frankel cite that in normal activities, a tendon is subjected to only about 25% of the ultimate stress that the tissue is capable of withstanding.[42] Research has clearly shown that the fifth day following an injury to a tendon appears to be when the tendon exhibits its weakest tensile strength properties.[5,16,41-42] After day 5, the tensile strength appears to progressively get stronger.

Since a tendon connects a muscle to a bone, it is subject to stresses any time a movement is performed, whether it be active or passive in nature. This should be considered during any phase of rehabilitation when a tendon is taking part in the healing process. Musculotendinous units work together very closely and can become taut during agonist as well as antagonist movements. For example, if a person has an injury to the quadriceps tendon, not only will active contractions of the quadriceps muscle group lead to discomfort via stress, so also may a contraction of the hamstring muscle group that subsequently puts the quadriceps tendon on stretch.

Ligament

A sprain to a ligament will present itself with inflammation and pain, as most ligaments in the body are high in neurovascular abundance. Complete healing of ligamentous tissue may take up to 2 years, and tensile strength may still be affected by a 30% to 50% deficit. Studies have shown that prolonged immobilization following ligament injury can lead to cell atrophy and thus increase the risk of rupture under stressful situations.[2,48] Furthermore, the lack of mobilization may decrease the rate of healing by not providing adequate nutrients to the healing tissue and influencing the collagen laydown in a biased formation. The laying down of tissue in a biased formation allows for greater tensile strength as the fibers become intertwined to form an increase in cross bridges. To the contrary, early mobilization allows not only for influential collagen laydown, but also provides nutrients for healing via the release of synovial fluid and increased circulation to the surrounding joints.

Frankel and Nordin[42] have identified three factors that influence ligament healing:

- Fiber orientation
- Properties of fibers
- Proportion of fibers

Fiber orientation of tendons are parallel, thus allowing for acceptance of high tensile loads. Skin, on the other hand, has a diverse orientation, allowing for high levels of extensibility. Ligaments fit somewhere in between, allowing for some extensibility, yet providing enough tensile strength to protect joint structures.[42]

The second factor is the properties of ligamentous tissue. Collagen and elastic fibers make up approximately 90% of the tissue. These fibers may influence the overall tensile strength of the tissue itself. Collagen is reported to be ductile, while elastic fibers are brittle.[42]

The third factor is the actual ratio or percentage of collagen fibers to elastic fibers. Ligaments are mainly collagen, and the strength is also related to the thickness and width of the fibers.[42] Yamada reports that elastic recovery in certain ligaments is as high as 99%, thus placing an emphasis on the importance of influencing the laydown of collagen components in a ligament during the rehabilitation phases.[47] The actual time frame of when ligaments are fully healed and revascularized remains unclear.

All ligaments in the body will heal at different rates depending on their physiological characteristics. In addition, if a ligament is torn to the extent in which its two disrupted ends have no possibility of connecting with one another, then there is an unlikelihood that approximation and full healing will occur. To promote optimal scar tissue formation during ligament healing, controlled stresses must also be placed on the tissue at hand. This process becomes slightly more delicate versus the stresses applied to muscle tissue since ligaments are not only very sensitive with respect to pain, but they also serve to provide protection to joints. Therefore, too much stress during any phase of healing can actually cause a disruption and/or separation of the healing tissue, thus leading to joint instability. This is especially true since the healing tissue does not possess the same original properties with respect to collagen extensibility. These

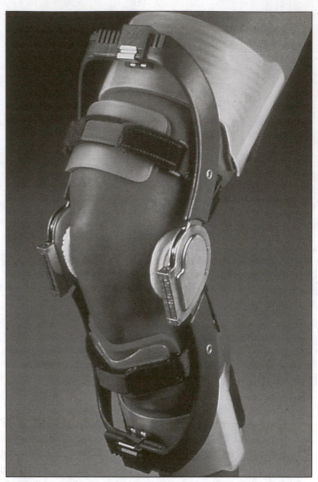

Figure 5-4. The use of a functional brace designed to restrict range of motion and protect healing tissue.

factors, in part, support the theory of using external orthotics or braces that restrict one's range of motion in an attempt to provide protection for the healing ligament and the related joint that it serves (Figure 5-4).

Cartilage

The majority of both articular cartilage and fibrocartilage lacks sufficient supplies of neurovascular accompaniment. Therefore, this type of tissue does not typically repair itself. Initially, as cartilage wears down through injury over a prolonged period of time, the tissue softens, a condition referred to as chondromalacia.[45] Traumatic injuries to cartilage can partially or completely tear tissue within seconds. These injuries do not lead to direct major inflammatory or pain responses since cartilaginous tissue is low in neurovascular supply. However, resultant pressure and/or damage to surrounding tissue such as underlying bones or nearby muscles may lead to the afore-mentioned responses.

When articular cartilage is damaged, it may not necessarily create pain or discomfort to an individual. It is not until the cartilage wears down far enough to allow for compressive forces to affect the subchondral part of the bone that discomfort occurs. An example of this is seen at the tibiofemoral joint, where forces are placed on the long axes of the tibia and femur on a daily basis. Over a prolonged period of time, and especially with highly repetitive compressive activities such as running, the articular cartilage will begin to destruct at both the femoral condyles and the tibial plateaus. Not until the cartilage has become softened and then destructed will the majority of pain be felt. Clinically, this would be a sign to a therapist that exercises to strengthen the surrounding structures should be performed in a non-stressful, or in this case nonweightbearing, manner.

Fibrocartilage can also be affected. While much thicker and resilient, it serves more as a shock absorber. However, it too can be injured in many ways. Like articular cartilage, when fibrocartilage is removed from its role, forces that would normally be dissipated by the fibrocartilage are now transferred to the adjacent bony surfaces. Again, in a weightbearing situation, this can become quite painful to an individual when performing resistance type activity. Unlike articular cartilage, there are small areas of some fibrocartilage that do have a very small vascular supply and can actually demonstrate healing capacity. Withstanding that exception, most injuries to fibrocartilage tissue remain as such, and typically the fibrocartilage is removed from the individual's joint surface since it sometimes leads to an abnormal end feel and restricted range of motion. When this occurs, the capacity to withstand forces via fibrocartilage that has decreased in size increases the amount of force per unit area. This will put more stress on the remaining fibrocartilage and ultimately lead to increased joint surface forces as well.

Nerve

Once a nerve cell dies, regeneration cannot occur. However, if a nerve fiber is disrupted, it does have the capability of regenerating and serves a better chance to regenerate the further it is away from the nerve cell. Peripheral nerve regeneration has been reported to occur at a rate of approximately 1 to 4 mm per day.[20,45] Basically, the less

involved the nerve fiber, the more rapidly it can potentially regenerate. With complete disruption of a nerve (neurotmesis), surgical repair is often indicated to approximate the ends of the nerve fibers in an attempt to facilitate healing and repair.[49,50]

Injury to a nerve that has resulted in a total disruption does not present with the typical types of pain that one experiences when various other tissue is injured. In fact, if a nerve is completely disrupted, sensation to the area that the specific nerve supplies will be absent. This is a clinical sign that one cannot overlook, as decreased or lack of sensation is a contraindication to many treatment techniques during the rehabilitation process. Some of these include the administration of thermal agents such as heat and cold, ultrasound, electrical stimulation, and the application of certain compressive devices.

Also seen with many nerve injuries is an inability to perform motor functions by the specific muscles being supplied by the involved nerve. Not being able to actively contract a muscle over a period of time may lead to adaptive shortening of a muscle, joint contracture, and muscle atrophy. Some of these side effects can be minimized with intervention of passive mobilization techniques that can restore normal length-tension ratios as well joint accessory motion.

Bone

The healing process of a fractured bone varies from that of the soft tissue structures previously mentioned. Healing of bone consists of five stages:

1. Hematoma formation
2. Cellular proliferation
3. Callus formation
4. Ossification
5. Remodeling[50]

Hematoma formation occurs during the first 48 to 72 hours. Dead bone and related soft tissue undergo an inflammatory reaction similar to that described earlier in this chapter. Granulation then occurs during the cellular proliferation stage, as the ends of the fractured bone attempt to form a fibrous junction. Initially, the unity is one of cartilage before it actually turns into bone structure. This will occur only after oxygen tension and compression are present in adequate amounts. Callus formation initially presents in a soft form until approximately 3 to 4 weeks, when it becomes hard in nature. Ossification occurs following adequate immobilization and compression, whereby strong bridges of callus assist in uniting the two ends. Remodeling, in which the stress lines of the fracture are strengthened, may take up to years to complete.

Optimal fracture healing is dependent upon many factors. Among these factors are a good blood supply, adequate immobilization during the early stages, proper stress and strain during the healing process, and support of the surrounding structures. Furthermore, the age, gender, and activity level of an individual, as well as the nutritional status of the host cells, will play an important role in the overall healing process.[47,52-53]

When a fractured bone is undergoing healing through immobilization, there are many activities that can be performed to maintain the cardiovascular endurance and musculoskeletal fitness levels of an individual. Shankman identifies the following rehabilitation goals during immobilization of healing fractures:[10]

1. Improve the overall fitness of the individual.
2. Promote range of motion of the unaffected, non-immobilized joints.
3. Minimize muscle atrophy.
4. Maintain or improve muscular strength.
5. Protect the healing structures.
6. Teach safe and effective transfers and gait activities.

PRACTICAL CONSIDERATIONS

The process of tissue healing and repair is quite complex. It involves many distinctly different phases that work together—at times simultaneously—at other times sequentially. While the overall process of healing tissue can be explained with respect to biochemical, vascular, and cellular changes that take place, there is still plenty of room for the unknown as the practicing clinician strives to achieve optimal biomechanics for each and every subject with which he or she works.

Even when analyzing a person with perfectly healthy tissue, it is quite common to observe less than ideal biomechanics at different joints. When working with injured tissue, the ability to restore normal mechanics may be at a slight disadvantage; therefore, it is imperative that the clinician have a sound understanding of not only normal mechanics for a specific type of tissue or tissues, but also the properties of that tissue and how it responds to injury.

As previously mentioned, different types of tissue heal in different ways. Even similar types of tissue can be influenced by many factors that may ultimately alter the outcome. The role of the clinician is to fully understand the healing principles with respect to an injury and the tissue that is involved. It is important to recognize that while tissues have been discussed here individually, many injuries will actually involve more than one type of tissue that has been damaged. With this in mind, one must be able to decipher through a plethora of information to come to a decision for optimal rehabilitation that is based on scientific principles and sound judgment.

The following is a list of considerations that a clinician should include prior to designing a program that will return a person back to premorbid levels of functioning following a tissue injury:

1. What type of tissue is involved?
2. To what extent is the damage?
3. What was the mechanism of injury?
4. Did it leave any underlying instability?
5. What are the healing properties of the tissue involved?
6. Is there an accompanying inflammatory response?
7. Does the tissue need to be protected via immobilization?
8. Is it safe to mobilize the tissue? How soon? How often?
9. What is the nutritional status of the tissue?
10. What are the subject's goals?
11. What is the activity level of the subject?

By no means is this list of considerations to be interpreted as all-inclusive. As a clinician, experience and intuitiveness must also weigh in the decision-making process. Therefore, even individuals who possess the same type of injury to similar tissue may be progressing at different rates through the healing phase. For this reason, it is important not to develop a strict regimen for a given injury without consideration of the above mentioned factors. Most importantly, one can only progress as fast as the weakest link will allow.

References

1. Houglum PA. Soft tissue healing and its impact on rehabilitation. *Journal of Sports Rehabilitation.* 1992; 1:19-39.
2. Andriacchi T, Sabiston P, DeHaven K, et al. Ligament: injury and repair. In: Woo SL-Y, Buckwalter JA, eds. *Injury and Repair of the Musculoskeletal Soft Tissues.* Park Ridge, Ill: AAOS; 1988.

3. Chvapil M, Koopman CF. Scar formation: physiology and pathological states. *Otolaryngol Clin North Am.* 1984; 17:265-272.

4. Christie AL. The tissue injury cycle and new advances toward its management in open wounds. *Journal of Athletic Training.* 1991; 26:274-277.

5. Dickinson A, Bennett KM. Therapeutic exercise. *Clin Sports Med.* 1985; 4:417-429.

6. Enwemeka CS. Inflammation, cellularity and fibrillogenesis in regenerating tendon: implications for tendon rehabilitation. *Phys Ther.* 1989; 69:816-825.

7. Gelberman R, An K-A, Banes A, Goldberg V. Tendon. In: Woo SL-Y, Buckwalter JA, eds. *Injury and Repair of the Musculoskeletal Soft Tissues.* Park Ridge, Ill: AAOS; 1988.

8. Hardy MA. The biology of scar formation. *Phys Ther.* 1989; 69(12):1014-1024.

9. Martinez-Hernandez A, Amenta PS. Basic concepts in wound healing. In: Buckwalter JA, Gordon SL, Leadbetter WB, eds. *Sports Induced Inflammation.* Park Ridge, Ill: AAOS; 1990.

10. Shankman GA. *Fundamental Orthopedic Management for the Physical Therapist Assistant.* St. Louis, Mo: Mosby; 1997.

11. Schurman DJ, Goodman SB, Smith RL. Inflammation and tissue repair. In: Leadbetter WB, Buckwalter JA, Gordon SL, eds. *Sports Induced Inflammation.* Park Ridge, Ill: AAOS; 1990.

12. Hertling D, Kessler RM. *Management of Common Musculoskeletal Disorders.* 3rd ed. Philadelphia, Pa: JB Lippincott; 1996.

13. Garrett WE. Muscle strain injuries: clinical and basic aspects. *Med Sci Sports Exerc.* 1990; 22:436-443.

14. Garrett WE, Lohnes J. Cellular and matrix response to mechanical injury at the myotendinous junction. In: Leadbetter WB, Buckwalter JA, Gordon SL, eds. *Sports Induced Inflammation.* Park Ridge, Ill: AAOS; 1990.

15. Garrett WE, Tidball J. Myotendinous junction: structure, function and failure. In: Woo SL-Y, Buckwalter JA, eds. *Injury and Repair of the Musculoskeletal Soft Tissue.* Park Ridge, Ill: AAOS; 1988.

16. Gillman T. On some aspects of collagen formation in localized repair and in diffuse fibrotic reactions to injury. In: Gould BS, ed. *Treatise on Collagen, Vol 2: Biology of Collagen.* New York, NY: Academic Press; 1968.

17. Kellett J. Acute soft tissue injuries—a review of the literature. *Med Sci Sports Exerc.* 1986; 18:489-500.

18. Lachman SM. *Soft Tissue Injuries in Sport.* St. Louis, Mo: Mosby; 1988.

19. Thibodeau GA, Patton KT. *Anatomy and Physiology.* 2nd ed. St. Louis, Mo: Mosby; 1993.

20. Arnheim DD, Prentice WE. *Principles of Athletic Training.* 9th ed. Chicago, Ill: Brown & Benchmark Publishers; 1997.

21. Stauber WT. Repair models and specific tissue responses in muscle injury. In: Leadbetter WB, Buckwalter JA, Gordon SL, eds. *Sports Induced Inflammation.* Park Ridge, Ill: AAOS; 1990.

22. Zarins B, Boyle J, Harris BA. Knee rehabilitation following arthroscopic meniscectomy. *Clin Orthop.* 1985; 198:36-42.

23. Kibler WB. Concepts in exercise rehabilitation of athletic injury. In: Leadbetter WB, Buckwalter JA, Gordon SL, eds. *Sports Induced Inflammation.* Park Ridge, Ill: AAOS; 1990.

24. Daly TJ. The repair phase of wound healing—reepithelization and contraction. In: Kloth LC, McCulloh JM, Feedar JH, eds. *Wound Healing: Alternatives in Management.* Philadelphia, Pa: FA Davis; 1990.

25. Hettinga DL. Inflammatory responses of synovial joint structures. In: Gould JA, ed. *Orthopaedic and Sports Physical Therapy.* St. Louis, Mo: Mosby; 1990.

26. Hunt TK, Van Winkle W. Wound healing. In: Heppenstall RB, ed. *Fracture Treatment and Healing.* Philadelphia, Pa: WB Saunders Company; 1980.

27. Zarro V. Mechanisms of inflammation and repair. In: Michlovitz SL, Wolf SL, eds. *Thermal Agents in Rehabilitation.* Philadelphia, Pa: FA Davis; 1986.

28. Odland G, Ross R. Human wound repair: epidermal regeneration. *J Cell Biol.* 1968; 39:135-151.

29. Werb A, Gordon S. Secretion of a specific collagenase by stimulated macrophages. *J Exp Med.* 1975; 142:346-360.

30. Tillman LJ, Cummings GS. Biological mechanisms of connective tissue mutability. In: Currier DP, Nelson RM, eds. *Dynamics of Human Biologic Tissues, Vol 8.* Philadelphia, Pa: FA Davis; 1992.

31. Madri JA. Inflammation and healing. In: Kissane JM, ed. *Anderson's Pathology, Vol 1.* 9th ed. St. Louis, Mo: Mosby; 1990.

32. Amiel D, Akeson WH, Hardwood FL, Frank CB. Stress deprivation effect on metabolic turnover of medial collateral ligament collagen. *Clin Orthop.* 1983; 172:25-270.

33. Farkas LG, McCain WG, Sweeny P, et al. An experimental study of the changes following silastic rod preparation of new tendon sheath and subsequent tendon grafting. *J Bone Joint Surg.* 1973; 55:149-1158.

34. Hooley CJ, Cohen RE. A model for the creep behavior of tendon. *Int J Biol Macromol.* 1979; 1:123-132.

35. Noyes FR. Functional properties of knee ligaments and alterations induced by immobilization. *Clin Orthop.* 1977; 123:210-239.

36. Porth CM. Cellular adaptation/injury and wound healing/repair. In: Porth CM, ed. *Pathophysiology.* 4th ed. Philadelphia, Pa: JB Lippincott; 1994.

37. Hernandez-Jaurequi P, Espereabsa-Garcia C, Gonzales-Angulo A. A morphology of the connective tissue grown in response to implanted silicone rubber: a light and electron microscope study. *Surgery.* 1974; 75:631-637.

38. Akeson WH, Amiel D, Woo SL-Y. Immobility effects on synovial joints. The pathomechanics of joint contractures. *Biorheology.* 1980; 17:95-110.

39. Forrester JC, Zederfeldt BH, Hayes TUL, Hunt TK. Tape closed and sutured wounds: A comparison by tensiometry and scanning electron microscopy. *Br J Surg.* 1970; 57:729-737.

40. Goldstein WN, Barmada R. Early mobilization of rabbit medial collateral ligament repairs: biologic and histologic studies. *Arch Phys Med Rehabil.* 1984; 65:239-242.

41. Hirsch G. Tensile properties during tendon healing. *Acta Orthop Scand Suppl.* 1974; 153:1.

42. Nordin M, Frankel VH. Biomechanics of collagenous tissue. In: Frankel VH, Nordin N, eds. *Basic Biomechanics of the Skeletal System.* Philadelphia, Pa: Lea & Febiger; 1980.

43. Kirscher CW, Speer DP. Microvascular changes in Dupuytren's contracture. *J Hand Surg.* 1984; 9A:58-62.

44. Prentice WE. The healing process and the pathophysiology of musculoskeletal injuries. In: Prentice WE, ed. *Rehabilitation Techniques in Sports Medicine.* 2nd ed. St. Louis, Mo: Mosby; 1994.

45. Athletic Training and Sports Medicine. Park Ridge, Ill: American Academy of Orthopaedic Surgeons; 1991.

46. Solomonow M, D'Ambrosia R. Biomechanics of muscle overuse injuries: a theoretical approach. *Clin Sports Med.* 1987; 6:241-257.

47. Yamada H. Mechanical properties of locomotor organs and tissues. In: Evans FG, ed. *Strength of Biologic Materials.* Baltimore, Md: Williams & Wilkins; 1970.

48. Kloth KC, McCulloh JM, Feedar JA. *Wound Healing: Alternatives in Management, Vol 5.* Philadelphia, Pa: FA Davis; 1990.

49. MacKinnon SE, Dellon AL. *Surgery of the Peripheral Nerve.* New York, NY: Thieme Medical Publishers; 1988.

50. Sunderland S. *Nerves and Nerve Injuries.* 2nd ed. New York, NY: Churchill Livingstone; 1978.

51. Gunta KE. Alterations in skeletal function: trauma and infection. In: Porth CM, ed. *Pathophysiology.* 4th ed. Philadelphia, Pa: JB Lippincott; 1994.

52. Churches AE, Howlett CR, Waldron KJ, Ward GW. The response of living bone to controlled time-varying loading: method and preliminary results. *J Biomech.* 1979; 12:35-45.

53. Frost HM. *An Introduction to Biomechanics.* Springfield, Ill: Charles C Thomas; 1967.

Suggested Reading

Alvarez OM. Wound healing. In: Fitzpatrick T, ed. *Dermatology in General Medicine.* 3rd ed. New York, NY: McGraw Hill; 1987.

Edwards CC, Chrisman OD. Articular cartilage. In: Albright JA, Brand RA, eds. *The Scientific Basis of Orthopedics.* New York, NY: Appleton-Century-Crofts; 1979.

Gelberman RH, Woo SL-Y, Cobb N. Flexor tendon healing: the effects of early passive mobilization. In: *Proceedings of the 27th Annual Orthopedic Research Society.* Chicago, Ill: Dependable Publishing Co; 1981.

Kloth CL, Miller KH. The inflammatory response. In: Kloth CL, McCulloh JM, Feedar JA, eds. *Wound Healing: Alternatives in Management.* Philadelphia, Pa: FA Davis; 1990.

Kumar V, Cotran RS, Robbins SL. Wound healing: repair, cell growth, regeneration, and wound healing. In: *Basic Pathology.* 5th ed. Philadelphia, Pa: WB Saunders; 1992.

Larocco M. Inflammation and immunity. In: Porth CM, ed. *Pathophysiology.* 4th ed. Philadelphia, Pa: JB Lippincott; 1994.

Levenson SM, Grever EF, Crowley LV, Oates JF, Rosen H. The healing of rat skin wounds. *Ann Surg.* 1965; 161:293-308.

Mason ML, Allen HS. The rate of healing of tendons: an experimental study of tensile strength. *Ann Surg.* 1941; 113:424-459.

Nordin M, Frankel VH. Biomechanics of whole bones and bone tissue. In: Frankel VH, Nordin M, eds. *Basic Biomechanics of the Skeletal System.* Philadelphia, Pa: Lea & Febiger; 1980.

Salter RB, Bell RS. The effect of continuous passive motion on the healing of partial thickness lacerations of the patellar tendon of the rabbit. *Proceedings of the 27th Annual Orthopedic Research Society.* Chicago, Ill: Dependable Publishing Co; 1981.

Tabary JC, Tabary C, Tardieu C. Physiological and structural changes in the cat's soleus muscle due to immobilization at different lengths by plaster casts. *J Physiol (Lond).* 1972; 224:231-244.

Tabary JC, Tardieu C, Tardieu G. Experimental rapid sarcomere loss with concomitant hypoextensibility. *Muscle Nerve.* 1981; 4:198-203.

Tipton CM, James SL, Mergner W. Influence of exercise on strength of medial collateral knee ligaments of dogs. *Am J Physiol.* 1970; 218:894-902.

Wahl LM, Wahl SM. Inflammation. In: Wahl J, ed. *Wound Healing.* Philadelphia, Pa: WB Saunders; 1992.

Worrel TW, NL Reynolds. Integrating physiologic and psychological paradigms into orthopaedic rehabilitation. *Orthop Clin North Am.* 1994; 3:269-290.

1. List the three phases of tissue healing and describe the main events that occur during each phase.

2. What are the clinical implications that need to be considered during each phase?

3. What are the specific healing principles that apply to each of the following tissues:
    a.   Muscle
    b.   Tendon
    c.   Ligament
    d.   Cartilage
    e.   Nerve
    f.   Bone

4. Based upon your readings, what are some of the considerations that you as a clinician would have when designing a rehabilitation program for a patient with the following conditions:
    a.   Acute medial collateral ligament sprain
    b.   Quadriceps muscle strain
    c.   Supraspinatus tendon inflammation
    d.   Colles fracture
    e.   Meniscal tear of the knee
    f.   Brachial plexus injury to the axillary nerve

STUDY QUESTIONS 5

CHAPTER 6

THE SHOULDER COMPLEX

Kirk M. Peck, MS, PT

OBJECTIVES

After completion of this chapter, the reader will be able to:

DIDACTIC

1. Describe basic anatomy of the shoulder complex.
2. List the motions occurring at the shoulder complex.
3. Describe shoulder girdle arthrokinematics and arthrokinetics.
4. Recognize the relationship of abnormal posture and mechanics of the shoulder to function.
5. Correlate various pathological conditions of the shoulder complex as they relate to functional anatomy.

PRACTICAL

1. Describe various force couples of the shoulder complex and relate their significance to normal shoulder function.
2. Discuss the implications poor posture has on functional anatomy of the shoulder complex.
3. Recognize the consequences that certain pathological conditions may impose on the normal function of the shoulder complex.
4. Describe the importance of concentric and eccentric muscle strengthening in shoulder rehabilitation programs.
5. Describe various rehabilitation concepts used to restore normal function of the shoulder complex.

OSTEOLOGY

Bony structures of the shoulder complex consist of the scapula, clavicle, and humerus (Figure 6-1). The scapulae are triangular shaped bones that glide over the rib cage through the interplay of several muscles. Each scapula is labeled by its borders (superior, medial or vertebral, and lateral or axillary) and its angles (superior, lateral, and inferior). These landmarks are often used to describe muscle attachments as well as common movements. Furthermore, the scapula has a number of distinctive prominences. Posteriorly, the spine of the scapula serves as a structure that divides the locations for both the supraspinatus and infraspinatus muscles. Anteriorly, an acromion process and a coracoid process are superficially palpable structures that serve as important sites for muscle attachments. The lateral angle of the scapula contains the glenoid fossa, which houses the glenoid labrum and the head of the humerus.

The clavicle runs from its medial end at the sternum to its lateral or acromial end. It provides the only direct attachment between the axial skeleton and the upper extremity. The clavicle is a long bone with a slight "S" shape.

The humerus is a long bone through which forces of the shoulder complex act upon.[1] The head of the humerus lies in the glenoid fossa, which is deepened by a fibrocartilaginous disc called the glenoid labrum. The head contains a greater and lesser tuberosity, which serve as common muscular attachments. Between these tuberosities lies a groove referred to as the bicipital, or intertubercular, groove. It is here that the long head of the biceps brachii tendon passes. Many other muscles also attach to the medial and lateral aspects of this groove. The shaft of the humerus also serves as an attachment site for muscles, such as the deltoid on the lateral upper one third. Distally, many structures of the humerus are specifically identified as common landmarks. These will be discussed in the next two chapters, as they serve more of a function at the elbow, hand, and wrist versus the shoulder complex.

LIGAMENTOUS STRUCTURES OF THE SHOULDER COMPLEX

Ligaments of the shoulder complex provide support during active and passive movements of

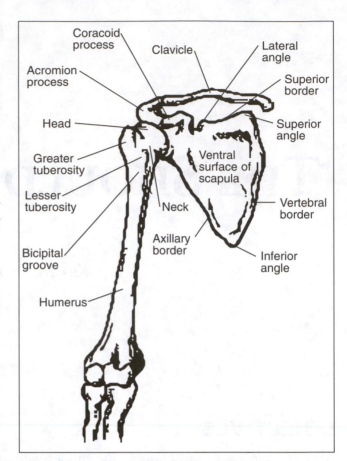

Figure 6-1. Osteology of the shoulder complex.

the upper extremity. With respect to the glenohumeral joint, it is comprised of a series of glenohumeral ligaments. On the anterior surface of the joint lies the anterior glenohumeral ligament, which can be subdivided into three broad bands. These bands are labeled the superior, middle, and inferior glenohumeral ligaments and serve to connect the humeral head to the glenoid fossa of the scapula. The anatomical relationship of this ligament helps to prevent anterior displacement of the humeral head from the glenoid fossa.[2] When the humerus is in an anatomical position, the superior portion is most taut, as opposed to full elevation in which the inferior glenohumeral ligament will then be taut. These ligaments also blend together to form the anterior capsule of the glenohumeral joint (Figure 6-2).

Posteriorly, the posterior capsule of the glenohumeral joint serves to assist in preventing a posterior displacement of the humeral head from the glenoid fossa. The coracohumeral ligament runs from the coracoid process to the anterior region of the greater tubercle and also assists in the anterior stability of the glenohumeral joint[2,3].

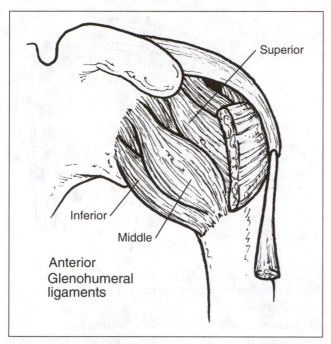

Figure 6-2. Anterior ligaments of the glenohumeral joint.

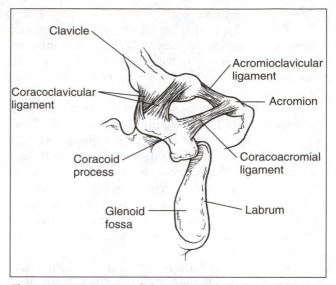

Figure 6-3. Ligaments of the acromioclavicular and coracoclavicular joints.

Ligaments protecting the superior portion of the shoulder complex include the coracoacromial, acromioclavicular, and coracoclavicular. The coracoacromial ligament runs from the lateral aspect of the coracoid process to the distal end of the acromion. It merely serves as a roof for the coracoacromial arch, as it is actually connected on both ends to the same bone. The acromioclavicular ligament attaches at the distal anterior portion of the acromion process and extends to the distal end of the clavicle.[3] The coracoclavicular ligament is actually composed of two separate ligaments known as the conoid ligament and the trapezoid ligament. These are more commonly referred to as the coracoclavicular ligament, which attaches on the superior surface of the coracoid process and extends to the inferior surface of the clavicle (Figure 6-3).

The costoclavicular, interclavicular, and sternoclavicular (anterior and posterior) ligaments provide stability to the sternoclavicular joint. Together, these ligaments provide dynamic stability for the upper extremity as the only attachment to the axial skeleton.[1] It is important to understand that any change in the extensibility of these ligaments, as in a tear or increased tightness, will ultimately affect the overall functional mobility and stability of the entire shoulder complex.

NERVE SUPPLY

Nerve supply to the muscles innervating the shoulder complex come primarily from the brachial plexus. This network of nerves, with additional contributions from cranial nerve XI and some lower cervical nerves, is responsible for providing both sensory and motor control for the shoulder complex. All shoulder movements receive innervation from one or more of the nerves comprising this network. Likewise, cutaneous sensory distribution is also provided by these nerves and other small cutaneous nerves. The reader is referred to the many anatomical references and suggested readings throughout this text for a more comprehensive look at the brachial plexus.

MUSCLES

Muscles of the shoulder complex are classified in many ways. Most commonly, muscles are classified by the action that they perform. For example, the subscapularis, latissimus dorsi, and teres major are considered to be internal rotators of the glenohumeral joint. Muscles may also be categorized by their innervation. This is a common way to identify muscular involvement when assessing pathology. For instance, the teres minor and deltoid muscle are innervated by the axillary nerve.

Knowing this, one can identify axillary nerve involvement by assessing these two muscles and their performance capability. Like other muscles surrounding a joint, muscles of the shoulder complex may also be referred to by their anatomical location, such as anterior versus posterior.

One common nickname given to a group of muscles around the glenohumeral joint is the *rotator cuff*. The rotator cuff is comprised of the supraspinatus, infraspinatus, teres minor, and subscapularis. While these muscles do not perform identical tasks, they all contribute to the rotational movement of the glenohumeral joint. Because of its proximity to these muscles, some consider the long head of the biceps brachii to be a rotator cuff muscle.

There are many muscles that assist with movement of the shoulder complex as a whole, as well as individual joints within the shoulder complex. Refer to anatomy texts and Appendix A, located at the end of this text, for a comprehensive review of muscle function about the shoulder. The majority of active muscular function occurs at the glenohumeral joint and the scapulothoracic joint, so we will pay special attention to the mechanics of these areas in future discussion.

JOINTS OF THE SHOULDER COMPLEX

The shoulder complex consists of articulations between the scapula and thoracic rib cage, the sternum and clavicle, the scapula and clavicle, and the scapula and humerus.[1] The scapulothoracic (ST) joint is generally not classified as a true joint but rather a unique articulation formed between the thoracic rib cage and the scapula via soft tissue and muscles. The ventral surface of the scapula is slightly concave with respect to a convex surface formed by the rib cage.[4] This relationship allows the scapula to glide smoothly over the ribs during upper extremity movements. Normal scapular dynamics are essential to the adequate positioning of the glenoid cavity during active shoulder movements such as flexion and abduction. Abnormal scapular mobility may inhibit adequate rotation of the scapula during overhead shoulder movements, which in turn may affect the quality of glenohumeral motion.[5,6]

The sternoclavicular (SC) joint is a saddle joint formed between the inferior portion of the proximal end of the clavicle and the superior and later-

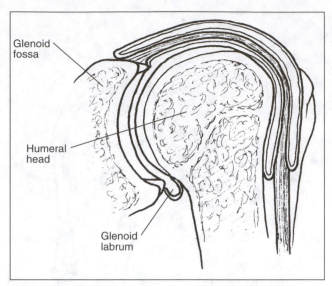

Figure 6-4. Glenoid fossa and labrum.

al portion of the manubrium. Lying between the two bones is an articular disk that absorbs shock and increases the contact surface area between the clavicle and manubrium. The SC joint provides the only direct linkage between the upper extremity and the chest cavity.[1]

The acromioclavicular (AC) joint is located at the distal end of the clavicle and is formed between the acromion process of the scapula and the clavicle itself. This joint provides indirect attachment of the scapula to the axial skeleton. Normal mobility at the AC joint, while minimal and difficult to measure clinically, is essential for efficient functioning of the glenohumeral joint.[1,4]

The glenohumeral joint is generally the most commonly thought of joint when discussing the shoulder complex. This ball-and-socket joint is formed between the glenoid fossa of the scapula and the head of the humerus. Reinforcement of the bony concavity of the glenoid fossa is provided by a thick layer of fibrocartilage, called the glenoid labrum. The glenoid labrum serves to deepen the fossa of the glenoid cavity, thus contributing to the stability of the humeral head within the cavity during glenohumeral movement[1,4,7,8] (Figure 6-4).

KINEMATIC MOTION

One of the hallmark characteristics of the shoulder complex is its diverse amount of mobility. Motions occurring at the scapulothoracic articulation include protraction, retraction, elevation, depression, and rotation. *Protraction* occurs when the medial border of the scapula moves away from

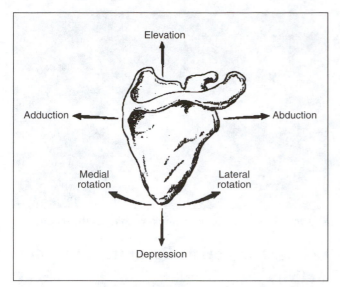

Figure 6-5. Scapular movement.

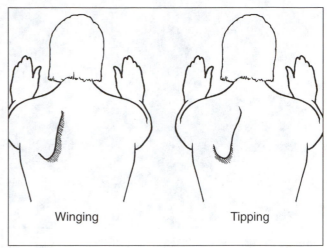

Figure 6-6. Scapular winging and tipping.

the spinous process and is also referred to as scapular abduction. *Retraction*, on the other hand, occurs when the medial border of the scapula moves toward the spinous process (scapular adduction). Scapular rotation may be defined in various ways by different authors. *Lateral rotation* occurs when the inferior angle of the scapula glides outward and away from the spinous processes, and *medial rotation* occurs when the inferior angle glides in a direction toward the spinous processes.[1] These movements are often called *upward rotation* and *downward rotation*, respectively. Once again, these movements contribute to overall shoulder function as can be seen in Figure 6-5.

The glenohumeral joint is generally considered to have 3° of freedom. Flexion and extension occur in the sagittal plane through a frontal axis. Abduction and adduction take place in a frontal plane around a sagittal axis, while medial (internal) and lateral (external) rotation occur in a transverse plane through a vertical axis. All of these movements are described with respect to the anatomical position. It should be noted that shoulder elevation often times occurs in the "plane of the scapula," which lies in an oblique plane and axis compared to those of anatomical position. Average ranges of motion at the glenohumeral joint are 180° of flexion and abduction, 30° of extension, and 80° to 90° of internal and external rotation. However, it should be noted that these motions will vary tremendously from individual to individual and may also be influenced by upper extremity dominance and type of activity. For example, over-head athletes will typically possess an increase in external rotation and a decrease in internal rotation.

Like the glenohumeral joint, the acromioclavicular joint also has three degrees of movement. The AC joint primarily permits scapular rotation in the frontal plane, but also allows scapular *winging* and *tipping* to occur.[1,5] In simplified terms, winging of the scapula refers to a posterior displacement of the medial border of the scapula. Tipping refers to a posterior displacement of the inferior angle of the scapula (Figure 6-6). Both winging and tipping of the scapula can alter the orientation of the glenoid fossa toward a more anterior or inferior position.[5,6] Changes in the orientation simultaneously change the position of the humeral head within the fossa itself. This dynamic change can lead to either an increased or decreased range of motion at the glenohumeral joint.

The sternoclavicular joint permits three degrees of motion to include protraction/retraction, elevation/depression, and rotation. Range of motion for protraction and retraction is approximately 15° in each direction. Protraction is seen as an anterior glide of the clavicle on the manubrium and retraction a posterior glide.[1,5] Adequate protraction and retraction of the SC joint enables one to achieve full scapulothoracic abduction and adduction respectively. Elevation and depression occur with simultaneous scapular elevation and depression. There is approximately 45° of elevation and 15° of depression available at the SC joint.[1] Rotation at this joint has been measured to be approximately 30° to 45° and also contributes particularly to shoulder abduction.

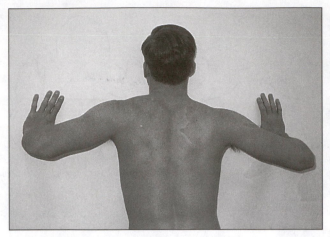

Figure 6-7. Push-up as a closed chain activity.

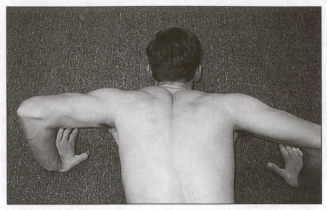

Figure 6-8. Push-up demonstrating winging of the scapula.

Open Versus Closed Chain Activities

Upper extremity movements are generally thought of as an open chain activity in which the distal end (hand) is free to move and the proximal (glenohumeral/scapulothoracic) components act as stabilizers.[1] Activities classified as open chain include movements in which one is reaching for or manipulating objects. Throwing a baseball is an example of an open chain activity in the upper extremity. In order to efficiently throw a ball, the hand must be free to move in space while the proximal shoulder muscles provide stability through strength and coordination. Weakness or fatigue in any of the scapulothoracic stabilizing muscles will affect the function at the glenohumeral joint and ultimately lead to shoulder pathology.[4-6]

Closed chain activities are less common at the shoulder joint. Such movements require that the distal end of the upper extremity be restrained from movement. An example of closed chain shoulder activity is a gymnast walking on his or her hands. This action requires an extraordinary amount of stability of the proximal shoulder muscles while the distal structures maintain contact with the surface of the ground. Performing push-ups is another example of a closed chain exercise (Figure 6-7). Closed chain activity of the upper extremity requires proper stability for optimal and safe function.[4-6]

Closed chain activities are possible only through the synergistic action of both scapulothoracic and spinal stabilizing muscles. For example, if weakness of the serratus anterior muscle is present during the performance of a push-up, then winging of the scapula may become quite visible to the observer[1,5,6] (Figure 6-8).

Concentric Versus Eccentric Shoulder Activity

Many examples exist to demonstrate functional applications of both concentric and eccentric muscle control of the shoulder complex. This can be seen quite clearly when one raises and lowers the arm in an attempt to grasp an object off a shelf. During shoulder elevation, the anterior deltoid muscle and, to a lesser extent, the serratus anterior muscle contract concentrically. Controlled lowering of the arm will cause the same muscles to contract eccentrically as they lengthen to a resting position. If either of these muscles possess insufficient eccentric strength, the arm will fall to the side of the individual with little or no control.[1,5] Since nearly all activities of the upper extremity involve both concentric and eccentric muscle contraction, these types of exercises should be incorporated into one's rehabilitation program when addressing muscular deficiencies and pathologies.

Active Versus Passive Insufficiency

Both the long head of the biceps brachii muscle and the long head of the triceps brachii muscle possess active and passive insufficiency as they cross two joints. Proximally, the long head of the biceps brachii is attached to the superior glenoid tubercle and the short head attaches to the coracoid process.[9] The crossing of the glenohumeral joint allows for the biceps brachii muscle to assist the deltoid with elevation of the humerus in the direction of flexion. When the elbow is fully flexed and the forearm is completely supinated, the amount of available force production from the biceps brachii muscle to assist with shoulder flexion will be limited as a result of an actively insufficient position.[5] One will not be able to efficiently use the biceps

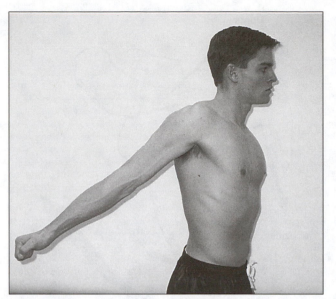

Figure 6-9. Passive insufficiency of the biceps brachii muscle.

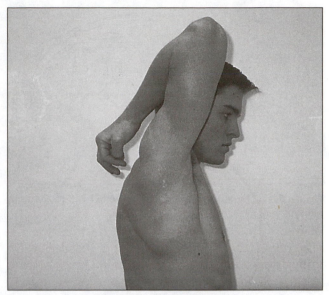

Figure 6-10. Passive insufficiency of the triceps muscle.

brachii muscle for shoulder flexion until the elbow is placed in a more extended position, allowing for synergistic contractions of the deltoids and the biceps brachii. Similarly, passive insufficiency of the biceps brachii may limit full range of motion during shoulder extension. If the elbow is placed in full extension while the forearm is maximally pronated, the degree of glenohumeral extension will be limited (Figure 6-9).

The long head of the triceps brachii may also demonstrate active insufficiency at the shoulder as it attempts to assist the posterior deltoid with glenohumeral extension. When the elbow is fully extended, the triceps brachii muscle becomes shortened and thus possesses a decreased force production with respect to shoulder extension. Passive insufficiency can be seen with the triceps brachii muscle when one attempts to perform shoulder flexion with simultaneous elbow flexion. The stretch placed on the triceps at its insertion on the olecranon process will limit active shoulder range of motion. Maximal shoulder flexion will only be possible if the elbow is allowed to fully extend (Figure 6-10).

Force Couples of the Shoulder Complex

Understanding the role of force couples about the shoulder complex is vital from a rehabilitation perspective. For example, during shoulder abduction, the humeral head is depressed within the glenoid fossa, preventing it from becoming compressed on the inferior surface of the acromion process.[1,4,5,9,10] Without adequate humeral head depression, rotator cuff pathology is inevitable. Stabilization of the humeral head within the glenoid fossa is made possible through concurrent contractions of the deltoid along with the rotator cuff muscles and the long head of the biceps brachii.[4,5,10,11] Abnormal function occurring in any of these muscles may lead to improper biomechanical actions. For example, a weak supraspinatus muscle with shoulder abduction allows the humeral head to excessively roll superiorly within the glenoid fossa, as opposed to inferiorly. This weakness leads to "impingement" of the soft tissue structures of the supraspinatus as it compresses into the undersurface of the acromion[10] (Figure 6-11).

Another very important force couple of the shoulder complex is seen with the upper trapezius, lower trapezius, and serratus anterior muscles as they move the scapula. During complete glenohumeral abduction, the scapula must laterally rotate to allow for the glenoid fossa to align itself in a more superior position.[1,5] Scapular rotation is accomplished as the upper trapezius pulls on the lateral aspect of the spine of the scapula, the lower trapezius pulls down the inferior and medial aspects of the scapular spine, and the serratus anterior creates a lateral and upward rotation of the scapula (Figure 6-12). By contrast, downward rotation of the scapula occurs through actions of the levator scapulae, rhomboids, and pectoralis minor muscles.[1,5,6] The levator scapulae act to elevate the scapulae while the rhomboids act to medi-

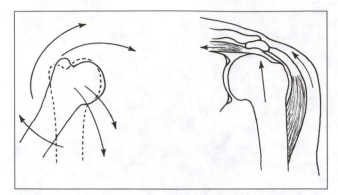

Figure 6-11. Normal and abnormal humeral head movement within the glenoid cavity.

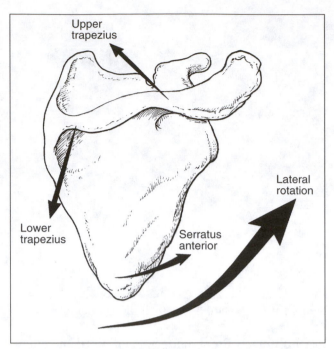

Figure 6-12. Force couple of the scapula.

ally rotate the inferior angle and the pectoralis minor serves to depress the scapula.[1,6]

SCAPULOHUMERAL RHYTHM

Scapulohumeral rhythm is a synchronous motion of both the scapula and the humerus, occurring during abduction of the arm. In simple terms, for every 2° of glenohumeral abduction, 1° of scapular lateral rotation is seen. This is referred to as a 2:1 ratio, whereby during a total of 180° of shoulder abduction, 120° come from the glenohumeral joint and 60° from the scapulothoracic joint[1,6] (Figure 6-13). It should be noted that the manner in which this movement occurs is not completely synchronous. For example, initially, more motion occurs at the glenohumeral joint as the scapula initially attempts to find a stabilizing position. Once the scapula has become comfortably stabilized, there is more of a 1:1 ratio occurring between the two joints' movement. Eventually, the scapula will once again establish a position of stability, and the remainder of the elevation will occur at the glenohumeral joint. Whenever scapulothoracic muscles appear to be restricted, full and complete glenohumeral motion will also be restricted. On the contrary, when the scapulothoracic stabilizing muscles are extensible greater than normal, or possess significant weakness, glenohumeral range of motion may be increased and ultimately lead to unstable positions of the glenohumeral joint.

Arthrokinematic Motion

Three types of movement occur at ball and socket joints such as the glenohumeral articula-

tion. These motions are rolls, glides, and spins. During shoulder flexion, the convex surface of the humeral head rolls in a superior direction in relation to the concave surface of the glenoid fossa.[1] In order for the humeral head to remain centered within the fossa itself, an inferior glide must occur. In the absence of an adequate glide, the humeral head will have a tendency to move toward the edge of the glenoid fossa, thus decreasing its stability. The spin component of the glenohumeral joint occurs during any rotational movement. During spin, the humeral head changes its point of contact in relation to a fixed point of contact on the glenoid fossa.[1]

COMMON INJURIES TO THE SHOULDER COMPLEX

Injuries to the shoulder complex are common in all populations. The various force couples acting to ensure proper function of the scapulohumeral region require synchronous movements of several muscles. Any deviation to these structures can lead to improper function and thus pathologic situations. The increased mobility that is seen at this joint makes it more susceptible to injury as well. Injury to muscles or joints of the shoulder complex are often accompanied by pain and functional impairment.

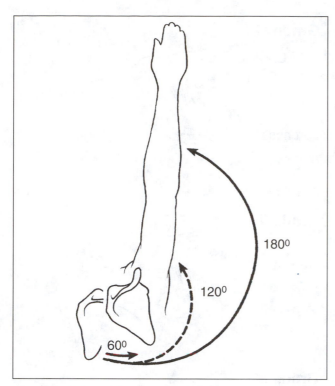

Figure 6-13. Scapulohumeral rhythm.

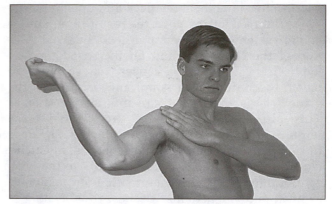

Figure 6-14. Mechanism of anterior dislocation.

Shoulder Dislocation

When one mentions a *shoulder dislocation*, he or she is referring to the glenohumeral joint. A dislocation to this joint is quite common since it has so much freedom to move. This large amount of mobility comes at a sacrifice to joint stability. The joint itself can become unstable or "lax" in a number of directions including inferior, anterior, and posterior. Inferior laxity involves a stretching or tearing of the superior portion of the joint capsule and surrounding ligaments, as can be seen in a traction type injury of the joint itself. Most commonly seen is an anterior dislocation whereby the humeral head translates excessively in the anterior direction away from the glenoid fossa. The mechanism of injury for this is a posterior force applied to the shoulder while the arm is abducted, extended, and externally rotated[8,11,13] (Figure 6-14). Depending on whether or not the humeral head remains displaced (dislocation) or reduces itself (subluxation) will determine the severity of the injury and one's ability to control the inherent instability. Posterior shoulder dislocations occur as a result of a posterior force to an arm flexed to approximately 90° in the sagittal plane. These are not as commonly seen but can be just as serious an injury as anterior dislocations. Rehabilitation of a dislocated shoulder includes a comprehensive pro-

gram to strengthen the rotator cuff and scapulothoracic muscles, and surgery may or may not be indicated.[13,14]

Shoulder Impingement

Shoulder impingement is a term often used to describe a variety of pathologies. By definition, an impingement is a result of a decrease in space that leads to structures compressing against one another. In the shoulder, this term refers to an irritation of the tendons of the rotator cuff and possibly the long head of the biceps brachii tendon as they pass under the acromion process in an area known as the subacromial space.[12] An impingement may occur when the humeral head is insufficiently stabilized within the glenoid fossa during active shoulder movements.[7,12,15] Dysfunction of the rotator cuff or long head of the biceps brachii may allow for excessive superior migration of the humeral head within the glenoid fossa. For example, weakness of the supraspinatus and/or infraspinatus muscles will reduce the normal amount of inferior glide of the humeral head within the glenoid cavity. During activities requiring shoulder elevation, a loss of inferior glide will cause the humeral head to roll superiorly within the glenoid cavity until it compresses upon the inferior surface of the acromion process. Due to their anatomical location, structures such as the subacromial bursa and the supraspinatus tendon may become entrapped between the humeral head and the acromion process, which can result in pathology such as bursitis or tendonitis.[12,13,16] Any decrease in the subacromial space as a result of inflammation, tendon fraying, bony anatomical malformations, or inadequate muscle functioning can lead to chronic cases of impingement.

Shoulder impingement may also be a result of

poor postural habits of the neck and upper extremities. Slumped sitting postures result in an anterior protrusion of the head and neck, internal rotation of the shoulders, and an increased thoracic kyphosis. This position causes the scapulae to medially rotate, which simultaneously forces the glenoid fossa to face a more inferior direction.[4,5] This altered positioning of the glenoid fossa impairs glenohumeral motion during shoulder flexion and abduction. As a consequence, repetitive elevation of the upper extremities above the horizontal plane will cause compression of the humeral head onto subacromial tissues, thus leading to an impingement of these structures. Rehabilitation of shoulder impingement pathology depends greatly upon the exact structures being impinged. Specific strengthening, stretching, and postural changes must occur in order to restore normal mechanical function of the entire shoulder complex.[5,17,18]

Shoulder Separation

A *separated shoulder* describes an injury to the acromioclavicular joint, specifically the ligaments of the joint itself. This type of injury is often the result of blunt trauma to the area and may entail a fall onto the shoulder or a blow to the shoulder, as when an individual gets tackled while playing football. A downward force to the tip of the shoulder will cause the acromion to pull away from the clavicle, resulting in a disruption of the normal ligamentous anatomy of this joint. Separation of the AC joint is classified as a grade I (mild), grade II (moderate), or grade III (severe) sprain depending on the severity of the injury[2,5,13] (Figure 6-15). AC separations will typically cause a great deal of pain and discomfort for an individual, particularly with overhead activities.

Rehabilitation for an AC joint separation may include temporary immobilization, followed by a gradual progression of range of motion exercises and eventually strengthening exercises to restore normal function. Surgical correction may be required if symptoms do not resolve with conservative care.[13]

Adhesive Capsulitis

Adhesive capsulitis, or *frozen shoulder*, is a term used to describe adaptive shortening of connective tissue surrounding and including the capsule of the glenohumeral joint. The anterior and inferior fibers of the capsule are generally found to

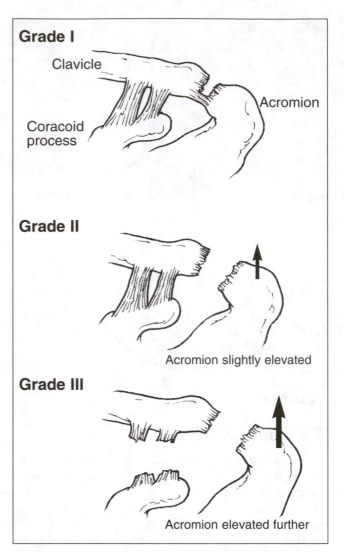

Figure 6-15. Grades of acromio-clavicular separation.

be the most restricted, leading to significant dysfunction of normal shoulder motion.[2,5] Typically, glenohumeral range of motion restrictions are most noted as one attempts to perform activities requiring external rotation, flexion, and abduction. Connective tissue tightness at the inferior portion of the joint capsule will force the head of the humerus to slide superiorly within the glenoid fossa.[13] The humeral head may then compress upon the inferior surface of the acromion process, resulting in an impingement of subacromial structures.

Clinical signs of adhesive capsulitis are most apparent when observing a subject elevating his arm overhead. A restriction in the glenohumeral joint capsule will require one to use excessive lateral rotation and elevation of the scapula to achieve the overhead reach. In addition, further substitution may be seen if inadequate functioning of the sternoclavicular and/or scapulothoracic joint is present as a result of disuse.[2,5]

Rehabilitation for adhesive capsulitis requires restoration of normal arthrokinematics of the glenohumeral joint and exercises to regain proper muscle balance in the shoulder complex.[13,17] One must be extra careful with the level of aggressive treatment for a condition such as adhesive capsulitis, as it is often a secondary pathology resulting from an underlying trauma. The classic scenario for development of adhesive capsulitis may involve a person who has traumatically torn his or her rotator cuff but has not received treatment for a couple of days to even weeks, for various reasons. Due to the intense pain associated with elevating the injured arm, and possibly an inability to elevate the arm at all, it remains at the person's side for a substantial period of time. It is during this time frame that the disuse of the arm leads to adaptive shortening of the fibers located at the inferior portion of the glenohumeral joint. Therefore, any treatment aimed at stretching or breaking up adhered fibers must consider underlying damage to other important structures of the shoulder complex.

References

1. Smith LK, Weiss EL, Lehmkukl LD. *Brunnstrom's Clinical Kinesiology.* 5th ed. Philadelphia, Pa; FA Davis; 1996.
2. Hertling D, Kessler RM. *Management of Common Musculoskeletal Disorders.* 3rd ed. Philadelphia, Pa; Lippincott; 1996.
3. O'Connell PR, Nuber GW, Mileski RA, Lautenschlager E. The contribution of the glenohumeral ligaments to anterior stability of the shoulder joint. *Am J Sports Med.* 1990; 18(6):579-584.
4. Culham H, Peat M. Functional anatomy of the shoulder complex. *J Orthop Sports Phys Ther.* 1993; 18(1):342-350.
5. Cailliet R. *Shoulder Pain.* 3rd ed. Philadelphia, Pa; FA Davis; 1991.
6. Paine RM, Voight M. The role of the scapula. *J Orthop Sports Phys Ther.* 1993; 18(1): 386-391.
7. Wilk KE, Arrigo A, Andrews JR. Current concepts: the stabilizing structures of the glenohumeral joint. *J Orthop Sports Phys Ther.* 1997; 25(6):364-379.
8. Wilk KE, Andrews JR, Arrigo CA. The physical examination of the glenohumeral joint: emphasis on the stabilizing structures. *J Orthop Sports Phys Ther.* 1997; 25(6):380-389.
9. Warner JP, McMahon PJ. The role of the long head of the biceps brachii in superior stability of the glenohumeral joint. *J Bone Joint Surg.* 1995; 77A(3):366-372.
10. Sharkey NA, Marder RA. The rotator cuff opposes superior translation of the humeral head. *Am J Sports Med.* 1995; 23(3):270-275.
11. Tsai Li, Wredmark T, Johansson C, Gibo K, Engstrom B. Tornqvist H. Shoulder function in patients with unoperated anterior shoulder instability. *Am J of Sports Med.* 1991; 19(5):469-473.
12. Kamkar A. Irrgang JJ, Whitney SL. Nonoperative management of secondary shoulder impingement syndrome. *J Orthop Sports Phys Ther.* 1993; 17(5):212-224.
13. Saidoff DC, McDonough AL. *Critical Pathways in Therapeutic Intervention, Upper Extremity.* St. Louis, Mo; Mosby; 1997.
14. Smith RL, Brunolli J. Shoulder kinesthesia after anterior glenohumeral joint dislocation. *Phys Ther.* 1989; 69(2):106-112.
15. Hjelm R, Draper C, Spencer S. Anterior-inferior capsular length insufficiency in the painful shoulder. *J Orthop Sports Phys Ther.* 1996; 23(3):216-222.
16. Zucherman J, Kummer FJ, Cuomo F, Simon J, Rosenblum S, Katz N. The influence of coracoacromial arch anatomy on rotator cuff tears. *Journal of Shoulder and Elbow Surgery.* 1992; 1(1):4-13.
17. Blackburn TA, McLeod WD, White B, Wofford L. EMG analysis of posterior rotator cuff exercises. *Athletic Training.* 1990; 25(1):40-45.
18. Cailliet R. *Soft Tissue Pain And Disability.* 2nd ed. Philadelphia, Pa; FA Davis; 1988.

Suggested Reading

Andrews JR, Wilk KE. *The Athlete's Shoulder.* New York, NY: Churchill Livingstone; 1993.

Carmick J. Clinical use of neuromuscular electrical stimulation for children with cerebral palsy. Part 2, upper extremity. *Phys Ther.* 1993; 73:514-522.

Hart D, Carmichael S. Biomechanics of the shoulder. *J Orthop Sports Phys Ther.* 1985; 6:229.

Inman VT, Suanders JB, Abbott LC. Observations on the function of the shoulder joint. *J Bone Joint Surg Am.* 1944; 26:1.

Kessel L, Watson M. The painful arc syndrome: clinical classification as a guide to management. *J Bone Joint Surg Br.* 1977; 59:166-172.

Matsen FA. Biomechanics of the shoulder. In: Frankel VH, Nordin M, eds. *Basic Biomechanics of The Skeletal System.* Philadelphia, Pa: Lea & Febiger; 1980.

McClure PW, Flowers KR. Treatment of limited shoulder motion: a case study based on biomechanical considerations. *Phys Ther.* 1992; 72:929-936.

Moreland J, Thomson MA. Efficacy of electromyelographic feedback compared with physical therapy for upper extremity function in patients following stroke: a research overview and meta-analysis. *Phys Ther.* 1994; 74:534-543.

Neer CS. Impingement lesions. Clin Orthop. 1983; 173:70-77.

Poppen N, Walker P. Normal and abnormal motion of the shoulder. *J Bone Joint Surg Am.* 1978; 58-A:195.

Saha AK. Dynamic stability of the glenohumeral joint. *Acta Orthop Scand.* 1971; 42:491.

1. Identify the osteology of the shoulder complex. Become familiar with common landmarks of each bone.

2. Using a skeleton, find the location of the major ligaments of the shoulder complex and explain the functional significance of each.

3. What are the major joints that make up the shoulder complex? What functional and accessory motion occurs at each?

4. How do open and closed kinetic chain activities of the shoulder differ? Does this have any effect on the surrounding muscle function?

5. Give an example of an activity in which a shoulder muscle may act both concentrically and eccentrically. How will a weakness or injury to this muscle affect the activity?

6. Demonstrate how a force couple works at the glenohumeral joint. What role does this play in preventing abnormal mechanics? Repeat for the scapulothoracic joint.

7. What is scapulohumeral rhythm? How can it be compromised?

8. Does posture play a role in maintaining proper shoulder mechanics? If so, how? What types of injuries can poor posture lead to?

9. How does normal shoulder mechanics affect overall function of the upper extremity?

10. Give an example of how a typical person might develop adhesive capsulitis of the shoulder.

CHAPTER 7

THE ELBOW COMPLEX

Julie A. Moyer Knowles, EdD, ATC, PT

OBJECTIVES

After completion of this chapter, the reader will be able to:

DIDACTIC

1. Describe and schematically identify the basic anatomy of the elbow complex.
2. Describe the function of these structures.
3. Using the rules of convexity and concavity, describe the joint motions that occur at the elbow complex.
4. Describe common elbow injuries and how biomechanics are associated with their treatment.

PRACTICAL

1. Palpate the distinguishing points of anatomy.
2. Demonstrate and be able to identify normal and abnormal ranges of motion.
3. Demonstrate closed and open chain exercises for flexion/extension and pronation/supination.
4. Demonstrate concentric and eccentric exercises for flexion/extension and pronation/supination.
5. Compare the end feels of flexion and extension and explain why they differ.
6. Measure the carrying angle and state whether it is within the normal range.

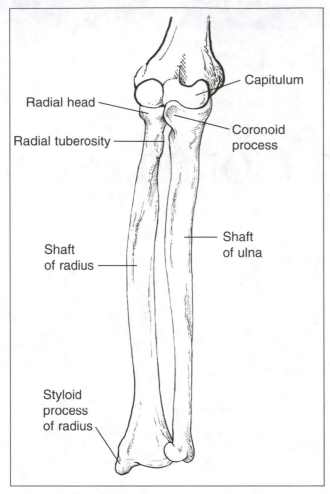

Figure 7-1a. Osteology of the elbow region.

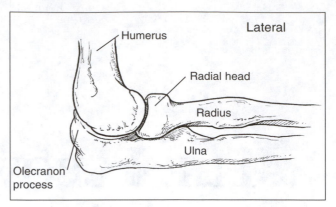

Figure 7-1b. Lateral view of the elbow complex.

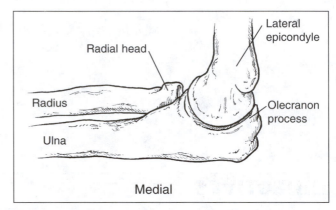

Figure 7-1c. Medial view of the elbow complex.

INTRODUCTION

The elbow complex is a very interesting structure located in the middle aspect of the upper extremity. Its position has defined its function: to connect the hand with the shoulder and the rest of the body. Without this connection, the mobility and function of the hand would be severely restricted. The elbow complex is comprised of several joints that are designed to promote the movement of the hand through space.

BASIC ANATOMY REVIEW

Osteology

The three bony components of the elbow are the humerus, the ulna, and the radius. The humerus articulates with both the radius and ulna, and the radius articulates with the ulna. The humerus, or upper arm bone, has unique anatomical features on its distal end. This anatomy allows the humerus to articulate with the ulna (humero-ulnar joint) and radius (humero-radial joint). These unique humeral features include a trochlea for motions with the ulna and a capitulum for motions with the radius. Between the capitulum and the trochlea is an indentation known as the coronoid fossa, and on the posterior aspect of the humerus is an indentation called the olecranon fossa. Next to the coronoid fossa is a third indentation called the radial fossa (Figure 7-1a through 7-1c).

The proximal end of the ulna has a "C" shaped concavity known as the trochlear notch. The uppermost tip of the trochlear notch is the olecranon process, and the bottom tip of the "C" is called the coronoid process. There is no radial notch on the lateral aspect of the ulna.

The proximal end of the radius has a concave head surrounded by a rim. On the medial side there is a concave ulnar notch with an articular disc at its lower ridge. The radius is much better developed at its distal end, as it plays an important role in wrist function.

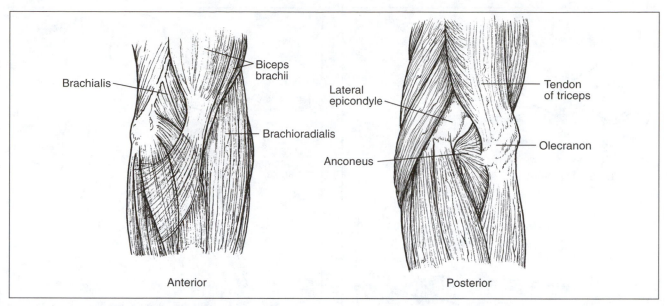

Figure 7-2. Muscles of the elbow complex.

Muscles

There are eight primary muscles associated with elbow motions (Figure 7-2). Two are extensors, three are flexors (one also supinates), two are pronators, and one is a supinator.

The triceps, which insert on the olecranon process of the ulna, is the main extensor of the elbow. The anconeus also extends the elbow. Since this muscle originates on the lateral epicondyle of the humerus and inserts on the olecranon process and ulnar shaft, it is not a very powerful elbow extensor.

The three elbow flexor muscles are the biceps brachii, brachialis, and brachioradialis. The brachialis inserts on the coronoid process and ulnar tuberosity, while the brachioradialis inserts on the styloid process of the radius. The biceps brachii, inserting on the radial tuberosity, is also considered a primary supinator based on this insertion. Furthermore, it is unique in that it has two origins: a long head and a short head. The long head actually crosses the glenohumeral joint, inserting on the supraglenoid tubercle of the humerus, thus assisting with shoulder flexion to a small degree. The other supinating muscle, called the supinator, originates on the humeral lateral epicondyle, supinator crest of the ulna and elbow ligaments, and inserts on the upper shaft of the radius.

The two pronators are the pronator teres and the pronator quadratus. The pronator teres originates at the medial epicondyle of the humerus and the coronoid process of the ulna. Its insertion is the radial shaft. The pronator quadratus, on the other hand, is a much smaller muscle, located further distally. It originates at the distal end of the ulnar shaft and inserts at the distal end of the radius.

Aside from these eight muscles, there are other muscles that originate in or about the elbow joint. However, most of these muscles play more of a functional role in the wrist and hand. The extrinsic wrist and finger extensors, for example, originate around the lateral epicondyle of the humerus. This is an area known as the *common extensor tendon*. The extrinsic flexors of the wrist and fingers originate around the medial epicondyle region of the humerus. This area is referred to as the *common flexor tendon*. These will be discussed in greater detail in Chapter 8.

Ligaments

There are four primary ligaments associated with the elbow complex. The annular ligament surrounds the radial head and connects it to the ulna at the radial notch. This ligament has an articular cartilage lining and also serves as a joint surface (Figure 7-3). When the radial head spins within the radial notch of the ulna, this ligament plays a role in stabilizing the joint.

The medial collateral ligament (or ulnar collateral ligament) is a very strong, triangular ligament that originates at the medial epicondyle of the humerus and inserts on the coronoid and olecranon processes of the ulna. This ligament helps to main-

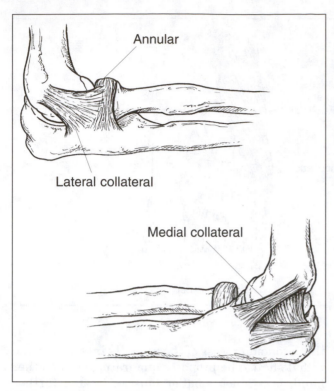

Figure 7-3. Ligaments of the elbow complex.

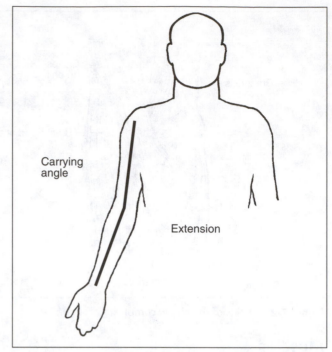

Figure 7-4. Carrying angle of the elbow.

tain humero-ulnar stability and acts as a checkrein for valgus stresses.

The medial collateral ligament, as well as all other medial capsular structures, is predisposed to additional stresses, unlike its lateral counterpart. These stresses are a result of what is known as the *carrying angle*. The axis for flexion and extension of the elbow is not fully perpendicular to the shaft of the humerus since the trochlea actually extends slightly more distally than the capitulum. During extension of the elbow with the forearm supinated, the outcome is actually slight lateral deviation of the forearm in relation to the humerus.[1] This angle, although reported to be up to 6 larger in females than males, varies slightly from individual to individual. The average range is documented to be between 5 and 19 [2-4] (Figure 7-4).

The lateral collateral ligament is shaped more like a fan. It originates at the lateral epicondyle of the humerus and inserts on the annular ligament and olecranon process. This ligament helps to maintain humero-radial stability and acts as a checkrein for varus stresses. Lastly, the oblique ligament, a cord-like structure, connects the proximal ulna (just below the radial notch) to the radius (just below the bicipital tuberosity).

Anatomy of the Nerves

Three major peripheral nerves pass through the elbow complex: the ulnar, median, and radial nerves. The ulnar nerve travels posterior to the medial epicondyle and is covered by a fibrous sheath that forms what is known as the cubital tunnel. Many refer to this superficial area as the funny bone. Injury to this nerve results not only in motor weakness to those forearm and hand muscles that it innervates, but also to the cutaneous distribution of the nerve on the ulnar border of the hand, the little finger, and the ulnar half of the fourth finger[5-6] (Figure 7-5).

The radial nerve is located on the lateral side of the elbow complex. It passes under the origin of the extensor carpi radialis brevis muscle and divides into deep and superficial branches. The deep branch provides major motor function to muscles involved with wrist and finger extension, as well as supination. Meanwhile, the superficial branch provides sensory functions to the dorsum of the wrist and the radial borders of the hand.

The median nerve is located centrally and can be found on the anterior surface deep in the cubital fossa. This nerve provides the primary motor function to the wrist flexors, as well as cutaneous distribution to the anterior aspect of the hand, first three fingers, and radial half of the fourth finger.

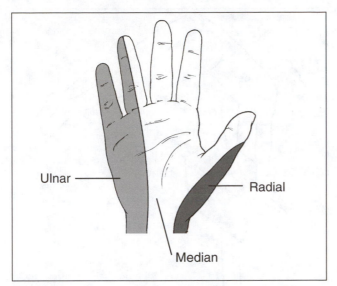

Figure 7-5. Cutaneous distribution of the ulnar, median, and radial nerves in the hand.

Miscellaneous Anatomy

A single, relatively large joint capsule surrounds both the humero-ulnar and humero-radial joints.[7-9] This capsule is reinforced on both sides by the medial and lateral collateral ligaments but is fairly free anteriorly and posteriorly. An interosseous membrane exists to connect the radius and ulna and provides additional stability to their combined motions both at the elbow and the wrist.

JOINT STRUCTURE OF THE ELBOW

Arthrokinematics

The elbow joints are comprised of the humerus articulating with the radius, the humerus articulating with the ulna, and the radius proximally articulating with the ulna. The radius also articulates distally with the ulna at the distal radio-ulnar joint. Centrally, the two bones are connected by an interosseous membrane. Although the elbow involves all of these joints, the commonly described *elbow joint* is actually the humerus and its articulations with the radius and ulna. These two articulations are typically addressed as one compound, uniaxial, diarthrodial joint, allowing for the hinged motions of flexion and extension.

The humero-ulnar motions occur as the trochlear notch of the ulna slides on the trochlea of the humerus. As the elbow proceeds into terminal extension, there is a bony end feel caused by the olecranon process of the ulna contacting the olecranon fossa of the humerus. On the other hand, active flexion of the elbow is usually terminated by soft tissue. Without soft tissue approximation in terminal flexion, the coronoid process of the ulna would come into contact with the coronoid fossa of the humerus.

The humero-radial motions occur by the concave head of the radius rotating with the convex capitulum of the humerus. As the elbow proceeds into terminal extension, no contact is found between the radius and humerus. On the other hand, in unrestricted flexion, the radial rim contacts the radial fossa of the humerus.

The proximal radio-ulnar joint (PRUJ), concurrently functioning with the distal radio-ulnar joint (DRUJ), promote forearm pronation and supination. During this motion, the radial rim, held within the annular ligament, rotates against the ulna. Meanwhile, the top of the radial head rotates on the capitulum.

Osteokinematics

Motions of the elbow are not only determined by the muscles that are contracting, but they are also dependent on the position of the elbow, shoulder, and forearm at the time of the contraction.

Elbow flexion and extension, occurring with motions at the humero-ulnar and humero-radial joints, have a normal range of motion of 0° to 145° to 150°.[10-15] Flexion occurs from three muscles that originate above the elbow joint proper and insert on the flexor aspect of the forearm below the joint. When these three muscles contract and shorten, they flex the hand up toward the shoulder. Since the biceps brachii originates above the anterior shoulder region and inserts below the elbow joint, it is the only one of the three flexor muscles that is considered a two-joint muscle; hence, shortening of this muscle also produces shoulder flexion.

Extension occurs primarily from the contraction of the triceps, and to a lesser extent, the anconeus. The triceps, as its name indicates, has three origins also known as *heads*. The long head of the triceps crosses the posterior shoulder region and together with the medial and lateral heads, inserts on the ulna just distal to the elbow joint. Hence, contraction of the triceps not only produces elbow extension, but also assists with shoulder extension.

Forearm pronation and supination, occurring with motions at the radio-ulnar joint, have a normal range of motion of 0° to 90° for pronation and 0° to 90° for supination. The starting position during measurement is with the elbow flexed at 90° and the thumb pointing upward. The forearm should be able to rotate 90° in each direction from this starting point. Thus, full pronation may be reached when the palm is faced downward and full supination reached with the palm facing upward.

Pronation and supination occur by muscles pulling the distal end of the radius over the ulna. With the exception of the biceps brachii (which acts as a supinator as well as a flexor), all other pronators and supinators are one-joint muscles and are not influenced by the position of the elbow in terms of flexion and extension.

OPEN AND CLOSED CHAIN ACTIVITIES

Open chain activities of daily living are common with the elbow complex. These include basic activities, such as combing the hair, to more advanced social activities, like throwing a baseball. There are, however, many activities that also require the elbow musculature to work in a closed chain format. For example, oftentimes floor installers and carpenters are on their hands and knees while working. Gymnasts are frequently in a closed chain upper extremity position and even wrestlers frequently attain this position (Figure 7-6).

Treatment for elbow injuries must therefore be adapted to the specific needs of the person. A tile installer may require faster speed open chain work to simulate the actual placement and movement of tiles, while also requiring higher load closed chain exercises to simulate the position of the hands and knees.

CONCENTRICS AND ECCENTRICS

Of all the elbow flexors, the biceps brachii is more commonly found to work eccentrically in a protective capacity. When the elbow moves quickly into an extended position with resistance, the biceps brachii works eccentrically to slow down the rate of elbow extension. A practical example of how

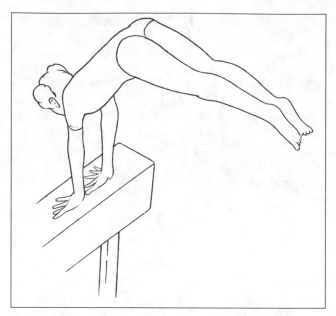

Figure 7-6. Gymnastics places stresses on the elbow joint in a closed chain position.

the biceps work can be seen as a person holding onto the top step of a ladder slips while climbing. With the hands grasping the top of the ladder and the body falling down, forcing the elbow into quick extension, the biceps contract while lengthening in order to slow down the rate of fall. The brachialis also works well eccentrically; however, it is much more effective when it contracts in the concentric mode.

The triceps is the major elbow extensor and works fairly frequently in an eccentric capacity. For example, during a push-up, the hands are fixed against the floor and the body moves up and down. The triceps are working in a closed kinematic chain. When the body is being pushed up, the elbows extend, the triceps shorten and perform a concentric contraction. When the body is slowly lowered toward the floor and the elbows flex, the triceps lengthen and perform an eccentric contraction so that the body may be lowered to the floor in a controlled fashion.

Active Insufficiency

The two-joint muscles that primarily influence the elbow complex are the biceps brachii and the triceps (long head). Consequently, these two muscles tend to be influenced more by active insufficiency. As stated previously, a muscle loses its ability to generate active tension if:

1. Maximum shortening has already been achieved; the muscle has shortened so much

that all of the cross bridges have been formed; and physiologically, myofilaments are unable to slide over one another any further.

2. The muscle is so lengthened that these myofilaments are unable to reach and overlap one another.

The biceps brachii becomes actively insufficient (shortened) when one moves into full elbow flexion while positioning the shoulder in full forward flexion (and the forearm supinated). It also becomes insufficient (lengthened) when the shoulder is in full extension, the elbow is in full extension, and the forearm is pronated.

The long head of the triceps becomes actively insufficient (shortened) when one moves into full elbow extension while positioning the shoulder in full extension. It also becomes insufficient (lengthened) when the shoulder and elbow are fully flexed. Changes in the length of these muscles should be a consideration of the clinician when designing a rehabilitation program aimed at restoring normal range of motion and strength as compared to the pre-injury levels of an individual.

Forces and Levers

The triceps move the elbow in a third-class lever manner. The triceps (effort arm), attached to the olecranon process of the ulna, are located distal to the joint axis. The humero-ulnar joint, located proximally, serves as a fulcrum, whereby the resistance arm then falls even more distal to the fulcrum.

The biceps brachii moves the elbow in a third-class lever manner. The biceps brachii is the effort force and is closer to the fulcrum or joint than the actual resistance arm (Figure 7-7). Both the triceps brachii and biceps brachii muscles are anatomically designed for range of motion versus strength and power.

COMMON ELBOW INJURIES

There are many biomechanically related injuries associated with the elbow joint. Elbow injuries are very popular in sports-related activities, especially during tennis and baseball seasons. Granna and Rashkin found that 58% of high school pitchers have elbow pain, 56% have radiographic abnormalities, and 4% have loose bodies.[16]

A common breakdown of elbow injuries in outpatient rehabilitation clinics is approximately 45%

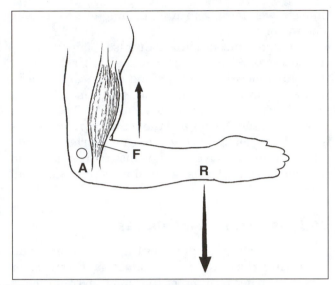

Figure 7-7. Third-class lever of the biceps muscle.

to 50% being related to overuse, another 40% to 45% falling in the category of valgus extension overload syndrome (including collateral ligament sprains and nerve-related injuries), and approximately 10% as miscellaneous.[17]

Epicondylitis of the Elbow

Lateral epicondylitis is an inflammatory response at the lateral epicondyle of the humerus, usually involving the wrist extensor muscles at their origin of attachment. Sports such as tennis, squash, and racquetball predispose large numbers of the population to the possibilities of this type of injury. The use of a racquet markedly increases the length of the force arm, or resistance arm, and subjects the elbow complex to greater stresses. The classic tennis elbow sign is caused by repeated forceful contractions usually involving the wrist extensors, especially the extensor carpi radialis muscles. Often times, tensile strength created at the origin of the wrist extensors can cause microtears, which lead to inflammation of the lateral epicondyle. The stress on the tendon may also cause small tears at the junction of the muscle and tendon and eventually result in tendonitis.

Usually those more prone to lateral epicondylitis have relatively inadequate strength, power, endurance, and flexibility of the wrist extensor muscles. This, combined with improper techniques and hitting a ball off center, can especially cause this problem. Thirty percent of expert male tennis players and 50% of expert females may develop lateral elbow problems, as compared to 75% of the general population. With the general population, muscle weakness and poor technique are usually the major factors.[18]

Medial epicondylitis can also be caused by these types of sport and work activities, usually forceful repetitive contractions of the flexor carpi radialis, pronator teres, and occasionally flexor carpi ulnaris.[19-20] These muscles are involved in the tennis serve, whereby the participant combines pronation, elbow extension, and wrist flexion. Many tennis players who incur this problem receive it from what is referred to as the "American twist serve."

Valgus Stress Syndromes

In various work and sporting events, especially during the acceleration phase of throwing or weightbearing position of the upper extremities, a valgus force is produced along the medial side of the elbow. This force stresses the medial flexor muscle mass and the ligaments located on the medial aspect of the elbow joint. As previously mentioned, an inherently large carrying angle may also contribute to an increase in medial elbow stresses. Concurrently, compression of the lateral side may occur as well. There can be actual stretching of the medial ligaments in either an acute disruption or a repetitive overload situation.[21] When the medial joint becomes unstable, stress is put on the ulnar nerve, the radial capitulum joint, and the olecranon fossa. Valgus extension overload syndrome (VEO syndrome) can slowly develop. Initially, there may only be vague pain along the medial side of the elbow, but if one continues to work or play without treatment intervention, more severe symptoms can occur.

In 1996, Brogden and Crow first described little leaguers suffering from elbow pain, swelling, and tenderness over the medial aspect of the elbow, usually associated with immature baseball pitchers.[22] Since then, the term "little league elbow" has been commonly used to refer to elbow injuries in young baseball players, usually pitchers, producing pain and tenderness especially on the medial humeral epicondyle region.[23] Biomechanical modifications, including the types and method of pitching, are recommended for individuals with these problems. Even the little league rules now specify how much rest and the number of innings a child is allowed to pitch in any one week. These rule changes are a direct effort to reduce the repetitive stresses placed on the skeletally immature anatomical structures.

Ulnar Nerve Pathology

Another common type of injury to the elbow is an ulnar nerve injury. This type of injury is not often seen until adulthood and is usually a result of a chronic irritation of the ulnar nerve. Sometimes the ulnar nerve will subluxate, or pop out of the cubital tunnel, as a result of a single stressor. If this occurs, worksite or sport modification may be necessary, and if still problematic, surgical anterior transposition of the ulnar nerve may be needed.[24]

References

1. Bowling RW, Rockar PA. The elbow complex. In: Gould JA, Davies GJ, eds. *Orthopaedic and Sports Physical Therapy.* St. Louis, Mo: CV Mosby; 1983.
2. Atkinson WB, Elftman H. The carrying angle of the human arm as a secondary sex characteristic. *Anat Rec.* 1945; 91:49.
3. Beals RK. The normal carrying angle of the elbow: a radiographic study of 442 patients. *Clin Orthop.* 1976; 119:194.
4. Steel FL, Tomlinson JD. The carrying angle in man. *J Anat.* 1958; 92:315.
5. Kisner C, Colby LA. *Therapeutic Exercise: Foundations and Techniques.* 3rd ed. Philadelphia, Pa: FA Davis; 1990.
6. Hollinshead WH, Rosse C. *Textbook of Anatomy.* 4th ed. New York, NY: Harper & Row; 1985.
8. Massie DL, Sager J, Spiker JC. Rehabilitation of the injured elbow. *Orthop Clin North Am.* 1994; 3(3):385-402.
9. Morrey BF. Anatomy of the elbow joint. In: Morrey BF, ed. *The Elbow and its Disorders.* Philadelphia, Pa: WB Saunders Company; 1985.
10. American Academy of Orthopedic Surgeons. Joint motion: methods of measuring and recording. American Academy of Orthopedic Surgeons. Chicago, Ill; 1965.
11. Clarkson MC, Gilewich GB. *Musculoskeletal Assessment: Joint Range of Motion and Manual Muscle Strength.* Baltimore, Md: Williams and Wilkins; 1989.
12. Hoppenfeld S. *Physical Examination of the Spine and Extremities.* New York, NY: Appleton and Lange; 1976.
13. Kapandji IA. *The Physiology of the Joints, Vol. 1.* Edinborough: Churchill Livingstone; 1970.
14. Kendall HO, McCreary EK. *Muscles: Testing and Function.* 3rd ed. Baltimore, Md: Williams and Wilkins; 1983.
15. Norkin CC, White DJ. *Measurement of Joint Motion: A Guide to Goniometry.* Philadelphia, Pa: FA Davis; 1985.
16. Grana WA, Rashkin A. Pitcher's elbow in adolescents. *Am J Sports Med.* 1980; 8(5):333-336.
17. Moyer JA. Unpublished data; 1997.
18. Nirschl RP, Sobel J. Conservative treatment of tennis elbow. *Physical and Sports Medicine.* 1981; 9:6.
19. Andrews JR, Whiteside JA. Common elbow problems in the athlete. *J Orthop Sport Phys Ther.* 1993; 17:289-295.
20. Youm Y. Biomechanical analysis of forearm pronation-supination in elbow flexion-extension. *J Biomech.* 1979; 12:245.
21. Cabrera JM, McCue FC. Nonosseous athletic injuries of the elbow, forearm and hand. *Clin Sports Med.* 1986; 5:681-700.
22. Brogden MD, Crow ME. Little leaguers elbow. *AJR Am J Roentgenol.* 1960; 83:671-675.
23. Pappas AN. Elbow problems associated with baseball during childhood and adolescence. *Clin Orthop.* 1982; 164:30-41.
24. Morrey BF. *The Elbow and Its Disorders.* Philadelphia, Pa: WB Saunders Company; 1985.

Suggested Reading

An KW. Morrey BF. Biomechanics of the elbow, In: Morrey BF, ed. *The Elbow and Its Disorders*. Philadelphia, Pa: WB Saunders Company; 1985.

Kessler R, Hertling D. *Management of Common Musculoskeletal Disorders*. New York, NY: Harper and Row; 1983.

London JT. Kinematics of the elbow. *J Bone Joint Surg*. 1981; 63A:529-535.

Parks JC. Overuse injuries of the elbow. In: Nicholas JA, Hershman EB, eds. *The Upper Extremity in Sports Medicine*. St. Louis, Mo: CV Mosby; 1990.

Tajima T. Functional anatomy of the elbow joint. In: Kashiwaji D, ed. *Elbow Joint*. Amsterdam: Elsevier; 1985.

Wilson FD, Andrews JR, Blackburn TA. Valgus extension overload in the pitching elbow. *Am J Sports Med*. 1983; 11:83-88.

1. List the joints that comprise the elbow complex.

2. After identifying the joints that comprise the elbow complex, isolate those bony articulations with respect to concavities and convexities.

3. Locate the major muscles surrounding the elbow complex and classify them as either flexors, extensors, pronators, or supinators.

4. What is the role of the following ligaments: Ulnar collateral? Annular?

5. Explain how the carrying angle of the elbow predisposes a person to medial joint stresses.

6. Demonstrate positions of the elbow that place the biceps brachii muscle in a position of active insufficiency. Repeat this for the triceps muscle.

7. What are some common activities that incorporate elbow function in a closed kinetic chain? Explain the role of surrounding musculature during these activities. Do they work in a concentric or eccentric mode?

8. Using the concepts of forces and levers, how would a person having difficulty overcoming a resistance during an elbow flexion exercise adapt or modify these approaches?

9. Physiologically, how do overuse injuries of the elbow differ in a child versus a skeletally mature adult?

CHAPTER 8

THE WRIST AND HAND COMPLEX

Jeff G. Konin, MEd, ATC, MPT

OBJECTIVES

After completion of this chapter, the reader will be able to:

DIDACTIC

1. Name the osseous structures that constitute the bones of the wrist and hand.
2. Identify the extrinsic and intrinsic muscles of the wrist and hand, and explain how they relate to function.
3. Understand the complexity of the ligamentous support in the wrist and hand.
4. Describe the arthrokinematic motion of the wrist and hand.
5. Define prehension and the different types of grip that are associated with function.
6. Describe the common injuries that occur to the wrist and hand.

PRACTICAL

1. Identify palpable surface anatomy landmarks as they relate to the wrist and hand.
2. Palpate the location of the various joints of the wrist and hand.
3. Actively and passively move the joints of the wrist and hand through anatomical ranges of motion.
4. Identify the limiting factors of wrist and hand range of motion in all directions.
5. Demonstrate active and passive insufficiency in the hand.
6. Demonstrate the biomechanical properties involved with various common injuries to the wrist and hand.
7. Demonstrate different methods of grasp.

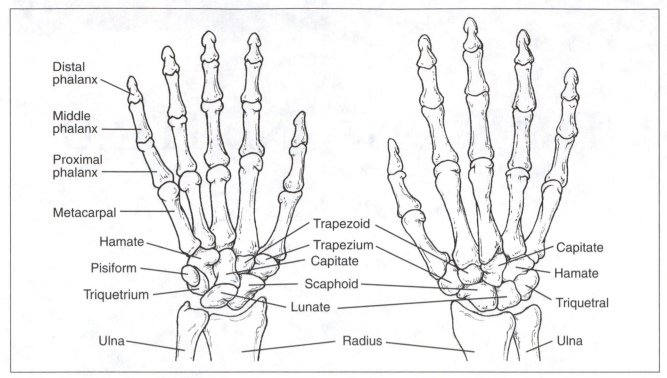

Distal
phalanx

Middle
phalanx

Proximal
phalanx

Metacarpal

Hamate

Pisiform

Triquetrium

Ulna

Trapezoid

Trapezium

Capitate

Scaphoid

Lunate

Radius

Capitate

Hamate

Triquetral

Ulna

Figure 8-1. Bones of the wrist and hand (palmar view).

BASIC ANATOMY REVIEW

Osseous Structures

The wrist and hand are unique parts of the body in that the tasks required to be performed at these locations range from using delicate fine motor skills to the recruitment of muscle fibers for forceful activity.

The wrist and hand area is composed of 29 bones that are organized in such a way that they form more than 20 joints. These bones consist of eight carpals, five metacarpals, 14 phalanges, the radius, and the ulna (Figure 8-1).

The eight carpal bones are aligned in two rows of four bones each. Proximally, they are bordered by the radius and the ulna, while distally they articulate with the metacarpals. The carpals are often referred to as irregular shaped bones, yet each claims its own unique configuration.

The carpals can be identified from the anatomical position beginning from the lateral aspect (radial) and moving medially (ulnar). The proximal row consists of the scaphoid, lunate, triquetrium, and pisiform. The pisiform, although considered part of the proximal row of carpals, is actually situated on the volar aspect of the triquetrium. The

distal row of carpals is comprised of the trapezium, trapezoid, capitate, and hamate. The hamate is especially unique in that it contains an extension that is described as a "hook" (see Figure 8-1).

Immediately distal to the carpal bones lie the metacarpals. As mentioned, there are five metacarpals, appropriately described as I through V, beginning with the first metacarpal on the radial side, located at the base of the thumb. Proximally, each metacarpal contains a base that articulates with one or more carpal bones. Each metacarpal also contains a shaft and a head, and the convex surface of the head further articulates with the respective proximal phalanx (see Figure 8-1).

Each hand contains 14 phalanges. Digits II through V each contain a proximal, middle, and distal phalange, while the thumb simply contains a proximal and distal phalange. The phalanges themselves are comprised of a base, a shaft, and a head.

Muscles

The muscles acting on the wrist and hand have been designed primarily to provide for a stable base of support while at the same time allowing for necessary and optimal length-tension adjustments.[1]

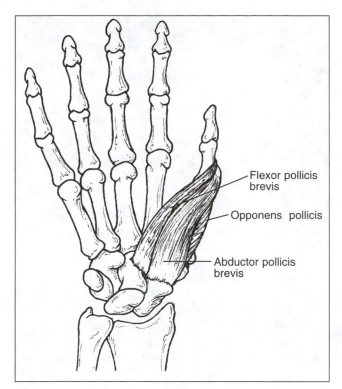

Figure 8-2. Muscles of the thenar eminence.

The classification of muscle function as it relates to the wrist and hand has previously been established according to different authors in a variety of methods. Soderberg relates muscle function to individual joint action.[2] According to this approach, examples of muscle groups acting at the wrist would be the wrist flexors, extensors, radial deviators (abductors), and ulnar deviators (adductors). Muscles may also be classified with respect to their position of anatomical location.[1] For example, the palmaris longus, flexor carpi radialis, flexor carpi ulnaris, flexor digitorum superficialis and profundus, and the flexor pollicus longus are all situated on the anterior aspect of the wrist and hand. These muscles are therefore referred to as *volar muscles.* By contrast, the extensor carpi radialis longus and brevis, extensor carpi ulnaris, extensor digitorum communis, extensor indicis, extensor digiti minimi, extensor pollicis longus, extensor pollicis brevis, and the abductor pollicis longus are all classified as *dorsal muscles* since they are located on the posterior surface of the wrist and hand.

Since all muscles are influenced by a neurological component, classification of muscles may also be done according to the nerve root level or actual peripheral nerve that a muscle is directly innervated by. For example, the flexor digitorum super-

ficialis and the flexor pollicis longus are both considered median nerve muscles since they are primarily innervated by the median nerve. Describing the muscle in terms of nerve root is slightly more difficult. Most muscles receive innervation from more than one individual root, and the contribution that is actually received from each level is not entirely clear. However, many sources will refer to a *primary root* as the major contributor to neural innervation for each muscle.[3-6]

Another method of classifying the muscles of the wrist and hand is by identifying divisions or compartments. The abductor pollicis brevis, flexor pollicis brevis, and the opponens pollicis are all muscles located in the thumb region that form what is called the *thenar eminence* or *compartment* (Figure 8-2), while the abductor digiti minimi, flexor digiti minimi, and the opponens digiti minimi form the hypothenar compartment on the ulnar aspect of the volar side of the hand. On the dorsum of the wrist, structures may be labeled in terms of the layer, zone, or even tunnel of which they appear to be a part.[4,6-8]

Lastly, muscles and their tendinous attachments can be classified as either intrinsic or extrinsic according to their relationship of proximal and distal attachments. Simply put, those muscles whose proximal and distal attachments are both found within the confines of the hand proper are said to be intrinsic in nature, while those muscles whose proximal attachments are found to be outside of the hand proper are said to be extrinsic in nature.

Ligaments

Ligaments of the wrist have been described by Whipple as being either intrinsic or extrinsic. Intrinsic ligaments appear to be very short and thin and most often connect neighboring carpal bones.[8] *Extrinsic* ligaments, on the other hand, appear flat and unimpressive, yet are able to form arches that assist with the structural design of the wrist and hand. As a general rule, the supporting ligaments that are found on the volar side of the wrist are larger and more extensive than those on the dorsum. Sennwald, et al have shown that the ligaments of the wrist help to coordinate the positioning of the carpal bones in the midrange of motion and help to restrict further motion of the carpals at extreme ranges of motion of the wrist.[9]

In the hand, palmar and dorsal ligaments and collateral ligaments combine with fascial extensions and capsular formations to provide stability

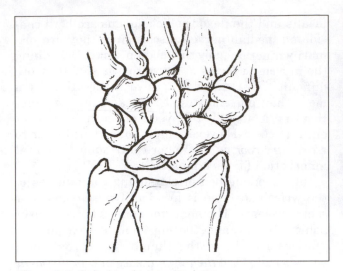

Figure 8-3. Radiocarpal joint articulation.

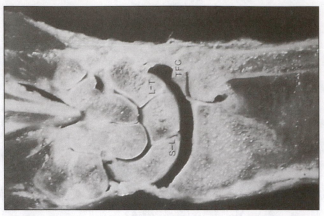

Figure 8-4. Ulnarcarpal joint demonstrating triangular fibro-cartilage complex.

in the form of passive restraints. Since the phalangeal region is a highly delicate, yet often stressed, area, the ligaments serve as vital components in the preservation of normal joint kinematics.

JOINT KINEMATICS

Wrist

It is believed that the radiocarpal, midcarpal, carpometacarpal, and metacarpalphalangeal joints all play a role in range of motion of the wrist. While each individual joint has unique functions, it is actually the total effort of all the joints that provides for optimal joint kinematics.

Radiocarpal Joint

The radiocarpal joint is considered to be condyloid in nature. It is formed by the concave surface of the radius and the convexity formed by the scaphoid and the lunate (Figure 8-3).

Two degrees of freedom exist at the radiocarpal joint. Typically, movement occurs as the carpals slide on the radius in a direction opposite of the movement itself. For example, during an extension movement, the carpals would move in an anterior direction. The opposite would hold true for a flexion movement, in that the carpal would slide posteriorly. Wrist flexion and extension primarily occur at the radiocarpal and midcarpal joints, and while a variety of studies have assessed the actual percentage of motion that each joint contributes, no clear values have been established.[10,11] There is

a consensus, however, that the radiocarpal joint contributes to a greater amount of flexion than does the midcarpal joint.

Radial and ulnar deviation also take place as a result of movement at the radial carpal joint. Here, the carpals continue to move in a direction opposite to that of the movement itself. With radial deviation, therefore, the carpals would move in an ulnar direction.

It is believed that the radiocarpal joint plays a significant role in ulnar deviation,[12,13] whereas its role in allowing radial deviation to occur is an end result of primary midcarpal joint motion.

At the radio-ulnar joint, the amount of available flexion and extension is often limited by soft tissue structures. With respect to ulnar and radial deviation, collateral ligaments play a major role in limiting available motion. In addition, the anatomically longer radius allows for greater range of motion to occur in an ulnar direction.

Ulnarcarpal Joint

While this joint does not possess a true articulation between the ulna and the triquetrium, it has been described in some literature to have some significance.[8,14-16] A meniscal type structure, referred to as the triangular fibrocartilage complex (TFCC), is situated between the distal ulna and the proximal part of the triquetrium (Figure 8-4). This area is sometimes called the ulnar-meniscal-triquetrium joint and acts in a similar way, as does the glenoid labrum of the shoulder and the menisci of the knee.

While movement at the ulnar-meniscal-triquetrial joint has not been clearly defined, the result of an injury to this region has been found to lead to instability of the wrist.[8]

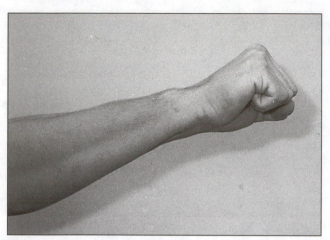

Figure 8-5a. Available range of motion at the carpometacarpal joints.

Midcarpal

The midcarpal joint is defined as the articulation of the proximal and distal rows of carpal bones. Unlike wrist flexion, it is believed that the midcarpal joint has a greater contribution to available wrist extension versus the radiocarpal joint.[17] As mentioned, the midcarpal joint also plays a greater role with respect to its contribution to radial deviation.

During wrist flexion, extension, radial deviation, and ulnar deviation, the center of the axis of rotation is believed to be located at the base of the capitate. However, it is important to remember that since these physiological motions occur as a result of the total accessory motion of each joint, the center of rotation may change as the joint angle changes.[13]

Carpometacarpal

As a unit, the carpometacarpal joint is formed by the articulation of the distal row of carpal bones and the base of the metacarpals. There are five distinct carpometacarpal joints that are considered to be synovial type joints. Each contains 1° of freedom in the direction of flexion and extension.

Separately, the second metacarpal articulates with the trapezoid, trapezium, and capitate. The third metacarpal articulates primarily with the capitate. The fourth metacarpal articulates essentially with the hamate. Physiological range of motion typically increases from the third through fifth carpometacarpal joints (Figure 8-5a). The second is fairly mobile, while the fifth has sometimes been described as actually having another degree of freedom in the form of abduction and adduc-

tion.[18] It is also believed that there may be some slight component of rotation involved that is available to allow for closure during the cupping motion.

The carpometacarpal joint of the thumb is formed by the first metacarpal and the trapezium. This joint is referred to as a *saddle joint*, having a thick but lax capsular surrounding. At this joint, flexion, extension, abduction, and adduction are key components that may combine with the movement of opposition to again maximize hand-cupping activity.

The primary function of these joints is to allow for proper formation of the arches in the hand. The combination of the small movements available at these joints, as well as the added support from palmar ligaments and fascia, provide for optimal surface contact utilized for cupping.

Metacarpalphalangeal Joints

The metacarpalphalangeal (MP) joints of the second through fifth digits are formed by the articulation of the convex head of the metacarpal and the concave base of the proximal phalanx. These are condyloid joints that allow for 2° of freedom in the directions of flexion, extension, abduction, and adduction. The latter two are evident during the spreading of the fingers, which is more prominent when these joints are in an extended position. This is a result of the tightening of the collateral structures as the joints move into a flexed position and provides for a more stable mechanism for gripping activities.[19] The joint also has a volar ligament that is firmly attached to the base of the proximal phalanx, which blends into the joint capsule and serves to reinforce the capsule itself.

The metacarpalphalangeal joint of the thumb is considered to be a hinge joint possessing one degree of freedom, flexion, and extension. It does not have as much available range of motion as do the second through fifth MP joints, but this motion is critical in function (Figure 8-5b). Both flexion and extension at this joint are key requirements of prehensile activities that will be discussed later in this chapter.

Interphalangeal Joints

Together, there are nine interphalangeal (IP) joints: one within the thumb and two for each of the other four digits. The IP joints of digits two through five are referred to as either the proximal interphalangeal (PIP) or the distal interphalangeal

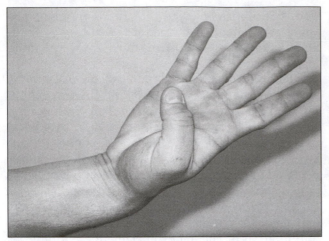

Figure 8-5b. Available range of motion at the first metacarpal-phalangeal joint.

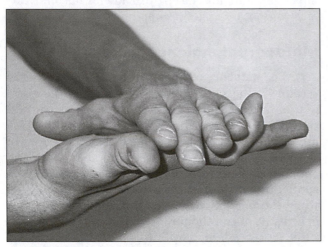

Figure 8-5d. Available range of motion at selected joints of the wrist and hand.

(DIP) joint with respect to their anatomical location. Each IP joint is a hinge joint with 1° of freedom allowing for flexion and extension to occur. In general, range of motion is slightly greater at the PIP joints as compared to the DIP joints (Figures 8-5c and 8-5d). As with the metacarpalphalangeal joints, range of motion also appears to increase as one moves in an ulnar direction. It is believed that this facilitates opposition by allowing the fourth and fifth digits to migrate closer to the thumb.

The stability of these joints is preserved by a capsule, a fibrocartilage plate, and collateral ligaments. These soft tissue structures along with the bony congruency serve as the limiting factors against excessive range of motion and/or instability at the IP joints.

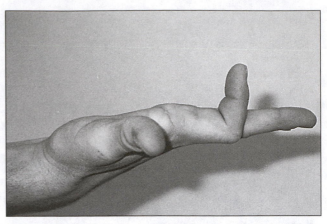

Figure 8-5c. Available range of motion at selected joints of the wrist and hand.

FORCES

Forces that occur to the wrist and hand area during static loads produced during activities of daily living have been found to be quite small.[20] However, during intense grasp, these joint-compressive forces may increase significantly. In fact, these excessive forces are transferred through the kinetic chain and can ultimately lead to structural failure.[10]

Of a more significant concern is when external forces are applied to the wrist. Injuries often result from a direct blow or stress that forces the wrist beyond its normal range of motion. This is the case when one falls on an outstretched hand (FOOSH) (Figure 8-6). While falling on an extended wrist applies a direct force to the area of the scaphoid, forces may be transmitted in the upward direction toward the lunate, the radius, and eventually the humerus. When the external force at any given point is greater than the body's ability to absorb these forces, a disruption will occur. This can result in contusions, fractures, strains, musculotendinous tears, or a combination of any of the these.

FUNCTIONAL POSITION

Many joints must work together to assume positions of function. Although this task is inherently reliable on the performance of muscles, ligaments, and joint movement, and is different from person to person, it has been determined that an optimal position does exist to allow for maximal amount of function combined with the minimal amount of effort.[1,17] This position includes (Figure 8-7):

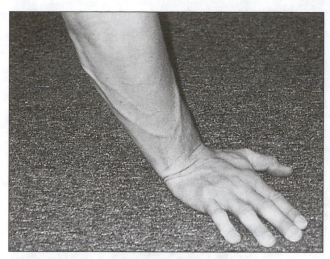

Figure 8-6. Fall on an outstretched hand.

- 20° of wrist extension
- 10° of ulnar deviation
- Slight flexion at the MP and IP joints of all digits
- Midrange opposition of the thumb

PREHENSION

The importance of being able to use the hand for the purposes of grasping and cupping has been discussed. This process is referred to as prehension. Since there are essentially numerous different methods that one can use to take hold of an object, the task of grasping objects has been divided into two components: *power grip* and *precision handling*.[21]

A power grip is typically used when the ultimate result is to forcefully grasp an object. This process involves the use of the finger flexors and possibly the thumb. A power grip has been described as a sequence of events:
- Opening the hand
- Positioning the fingers
- The fingers closing on the object
- Maintaining a forceful grip[22]

Traditionally, power grips have been measured clinically with hand-held dynamometers.[23] For purposes of classification, the power grip has been further subdivided into four types:
- A cylindrical grip
- A spherical grip
- A hook grip
- A lateral prehension grip

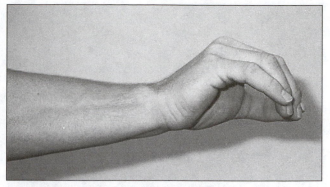

Figure 8-7. Functional position of the hand.

A cylindrical grip involves the grasping of an object by dynamic control of primarily the flexor digitorum profundus and flexor pollicis longus, but also with possible assistance from the flexor digitorum superficialis and the interossei.[24,25] This type of grip is often seen when one holds a glass of soda (Figure 8-8a).

It is sometimes difficult to differentiate between a cylindrical and a spherical grip. The main distinction between the two is usually a result of the size of the object. With a larger sized object, a spherical grip is utilized. Increased distances between the fingers are formed in an attempt to completely grasp the object (Figure 8-8b). In turn, one must rely more so on the actions of the finger abductors and adductors to provide a balanced contraction while the finger flexors continue to act. Holding a tennis ball is an example of using a spherical grip.

A hook grip is also similar to a cylindrical grip with the exception that the thumb is not included in this type of grip. The flexor digitorum profundus and superficialis are the primary muscles involved, and they may act independently or in conjunction with one another depending on the position of the object. Carrying a briefcase is an example of a hook grip (Figure 8-8c).

The final type of power grip is referred to as a lateral prehension grip. While this type of grip also involves the finger abductors and adductors, it does not utilize finger flexors. The primary muscles involved here are the interossei, although the finger extensors (extensor digitorum communis and lumbricales) play a role in keeping the fingers extended, thus allowing for greater force output of the interossei. Lateral prehension is seen at either the MP or IP joints and is performed by adjacent fingers. Holding a cigarette is one of the most common tasks that involve a lateral prehension grip (Figure 8-8d).

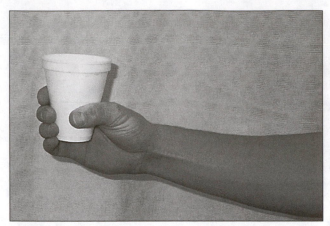

Figure 8-8a. Example of power grip: cylindrical.

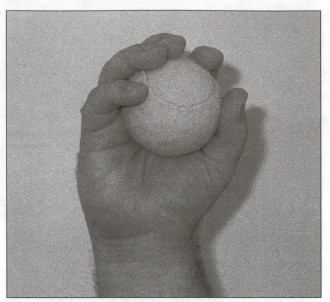

Figure 8-8b. Example of power grip: spherical.

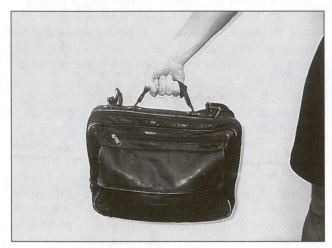

Figure 8-8c. Example of power grip: hook.

Precision Handling

While forms of precision handling may involve similar muscles to that of power grip prehension techniques, this is more of a delicate task that involves precise manipulation as opposed to forceful grasp. Proper fine motor skills, as well as adequate sensation, are essential for precision handling techniques. Three types of precision handling have been described as:

- pad-to-pad
- tip-to-tip
- lateral pinch

PAD-TO-PAD

The majority of precision handling occurs in a palmar pad-to-pad method.[26] This involves grasping an object between the pad of the thumb and the pad of another finger. Either the flexor digitorum profundus or superficialis may be involved, with the flexor pollicis longus and brevis, opponens pol-

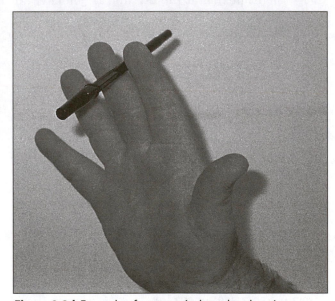

Figure 8-8d. Example of power grip: lateral prehension.

licis, and abductor pollicis brevis of the thumb. Examples of pad-to-pad precision handling is when one grasps a pencil, or the method in which one holds a dart (Figure 8-9). Pad-to-pad precision handling is difficult to perform following a median nerve injury due to the paralysis of the thumb muscles.

TIP-TO-TIP

Tip-to-tip precision handling is by far the most difficult to perform and possibly the most frustrating following injury to any of the structures involved. This is usually performed when handling very small or fine objects such as the activity of

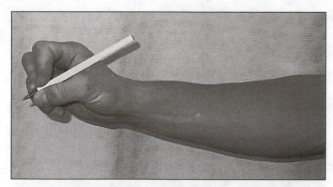

Figure 8-9. Example of pad-to-pad precision handling.

threading a needle. Again, the distal flexor muscles are very important for grasping and controlling the object, and additional MP (and specifically IP) flexion may be required to adequately maintain a functional grasp of the smaller object.

LATERAL PINCH

A lateral pinch grip can be seen when one holds a key. Here, the volar pad of the thumb is used to grasp along with the lateral or radial side of the index finger along the proximal, middle, or distal phalanx. This is not a very precise form of prehension but is often used by those who may have paralysis resulting in the loss of motor function of the finger flexors.

Essential Requirements for Efficient Prehensile Functions

Although different methods exist to provide for adequate prehension, it is believed that the following components are required to be able to perform prehensile functions efficiently:

1. Mobility of the CMC joint of the thumb and the MCP of digits IV and V to allow for peripheral mobility.
2. Selective rigidity of the CMC joints of digits II and III to allow for central stability.
3. Stability of the arches of all of the digits to provide for adequate cupping of the hand.
4. A synergistic and antagonistic muscular balance between both the extrinsic and intrinsic groups to allow for optimal length-tension relationships.
5. Adequate sensory function within the entire hand area for receptive fine motor skills.

ACTIVE VERSUS PASSIVE INSUFFICIENCY

As described in earlier chapters, the wrist also has a length-tension component that enables primarily the wrist flexors and extensors to work in a manner that would provide for sufficient grasp. Lehmkuhl and Smith note that a direct relationship exists between the effort of one's grip and the contraction of the wrist extensors.[19] That is, the stronger the grip, the stronger the contraction of the wrist extensors.

As the fingers move into a position of increased flexion, the wrist extensor muscles begin to activate to maintain the wrist in a position of extension while the fingers flex. You will notice that when you make a fist, your fingers flex into your hand. When performing gripping type activities with a fist-like grip, you will also notice that your wrist feels more stabilized while it is in a position of extension versus flexion. This is due to the fact that as the wrist flexes while the fingers are already flexed, the finger flexors lose their optimal length-tension relationships.

If you were to position your wrist into full flexion and then attempt to make a fist by flexing your fingers as well, you may find it difficult to close your fist completely. This occurs since the extensor tendons have fully elongated and therefore prevent the finger flexors from elongating any further. This phenomenon is referred to as *passive insufficiency* of the wrist (Figure 8-10).

Likewise, as the wrist increases into a further flexed position, you will notice that the finger flexor muscles become inefficient in producing stronger contractions. This is due to the ineffective tension developed within the finger flexors and results in a weaker grip, known as *active insufficiency*. It has also been shown that placing the wrist in a more ulnar deviated position may increase finger flexor force.[27] Therefore, performing grasping activities while the wrist is radially deviated may contribute to active insufficiency.

The mechanism for actually using active and passive insufficiency to enhance function is referred to as *tenodesis*. For example, a person may not have complete use of his or her finger flexors due to a neurological injury that has affected the median nerve. Does this mean that he or she may

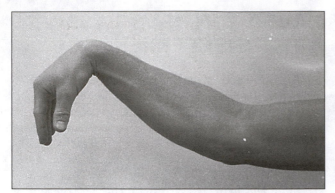

Figure 8-10. Demonstration of passive insufficiency of the wrist.

not be able to perform prehensile tasks? Not necessarily. Remember that extending the wrist places the finger flexors in a more flexed position in which they will move closer to the palm. This activity is commonly used by those who have had similar nerve injuries and require the use of their finger flexors for grasping objects as well as to perform transfers (Figure 8-11).

INJURIES TO THE WRIST AND HAND

Injuries to the wrist and hand have been reported as approximately 28.6% of all injuries treated in emergency rooms.[28] The mechanism of injury can be widespread, but the ability of one to function with the necessary skills becomes similarly difficult based on the nature and severity of the injury itself.

Traumatic Injuries

Most traumatic injuries to the wrist and hand region occur as a result of falls. Since most of us use our hands in an attempt to break a fall, this area becomes quite vulnerable to external forces. While none of us are immune to falls, the elderly tend to be at a greater risk, possibly due to decreased strength and proprioception[29] (Figure 8-12).

The most common form of protection from a fall is to land on an outstretched hand. This gesture places a tremendous amount of force on the scaphoid bone, explaining why it is the carpal bone most often fractured. The scaphoid, being as small as it is, is typically unable to accommodate all of the external forces that are applied to it during a fall. In the body's attempt to disperse these forces, the lunate, radius, and humerus follow a kinetic

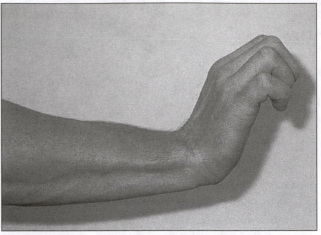

Figure 8-11. Person with deficient wrist flexors using the tenodesis method.

link in which each also becomes vulnerable to injury.[10] Fractures tend to be the most commonly seen type of injury to the wrist.[28] Fractures to the scaphoid are often noticed upon palpation in the area of the "anatomical snuff box," which is bordered by the tendons from the abductor pollicis brevis and the extensor pollicis brevis on the radial side and the extensor pollicis longus on the ulnar side (Figure 8-13).

Ligaments of the wrist and hand are injured quite often from excessive forces when a joint is placed into extreme ranges of motion beyond its normal capability. Since the ligamentous structures act to stabilize a joint, any tear to a ligament, minor or major, may lead to instability of the involved joint. An example of this is a tear to the ulnar collateral ligament of the thumb. This ligament becomes stressed when excessive forces are applied to the thumb, pushing into a position of extreme abduction (Figure 8-14).

The lay term for this injury is *gamekeeper's* or *skier's thumb*, as it is seen quite often within the population of athletes who frequently use the thenar muscles as an active force to grasp an object. A person with a ligamentous injury may return back to daily activities with the aid of a fabricated splint.[30-32]

Tendon Injuries

Injuries to the tendons of the wrist and hand occur fairly frequently and can immensely impact function. Tendinous injuries can range from mild inflammatory responses (tendonitis) to more severe lacerations requiring surgery and hospital admission.[28]

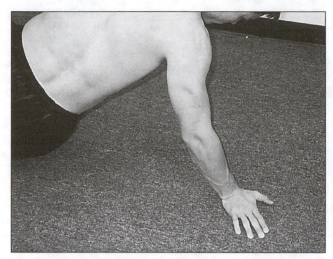

Figure 8-12. Using the extended wrist to break a fall.

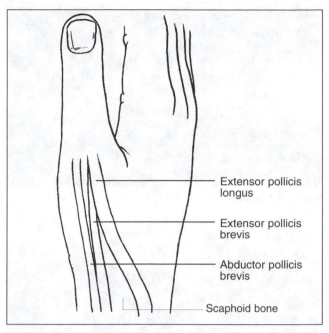

Figure 8-13. Anatomical snuff box.

Labels on figure: Extensor pollicis longus; Extensor pollicis brevis; Abductor pollicis brevis; Scaphoid bone

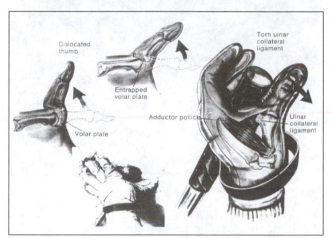

Figure 8-14. Skier's thumb (reprinted with permission from Kuland DN. *The Injured Athlete*. Philadelphia, Pa: Lippincott Williams & Wilkins; 1988).

MALLET FINGER

A disruption of the extensor digitorum communis tendon at the distal interphalangeal (DIP) is called a mallet finger (Figures 8-15 a and 8-15b). This occurs as a result of blunt trauma to the tip of the dorsal extensor surface, which leaves one with the inability to actively extend the DIP joint of the involved digit. The joint will still be able to passively extend and will require an approximation of the disrupted tendon to its attachment to enable adequate healing to take place. Occasionally, this may re-attach without surgery, but most often surgical intervention is necessary to regain normal function. Surgery involves sewing the tendon back to the distal phalanx.

JERSEY FINGER

A jersey finger is similar to a mallet finger in that the distal phalanx is unable to be actively moved. In this case, however, it is the flexor digitorum profundus tendon that has been disrupted and active flexion of the DIP that is lacking. The mechanism of injury occurs when one is pulling forcefully with the tip of the volar pad of the distal phalanx, such that is seen when a football player attempts to tackle an opponent by the jersey. If the opposing force is too strong, it will cause a tear in the flexor tendon. Management for this condition is also similar to that of a mallet finger. Extra care is taken with this type of injury to prevent the torn tendon from migrating proximally within the palm of the hand.

BOUTONNIERE DEFORMITY

This is a deformity resulting in abnormal extension of the MP and DIP joints in addition to flexion of the PIP joint (Figures 8-16a and 8-16b). Typically, this occurs following blunt trauma to the central slip of the extensor digitorum communis tendon, which is part of the extensor hood. A boutonniere deformity may also be present in those who have rheumatoid arthritis, as a secondary result of the deterioration of the synovial lining. This type of deformity is often treated with splinting to help restore normal alignment.

RHEUMATOID ARTHRITIS

Rheumatoid arthritis is a condition that commonly affects both the wrist and hand bilaterally.[33] The nature of the disease leads to a deterioration of both the tendons and the sheaths that surround

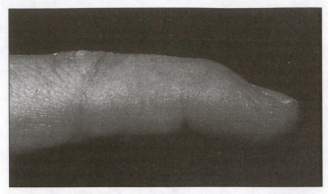

Figure 8-15a. Mallet finger.

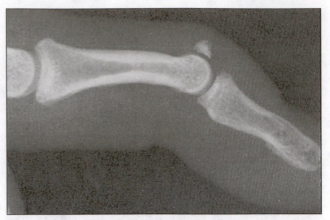

Figure 8-15b. Mallet finger with an avulsed fragment at the base of the distal phalanx.

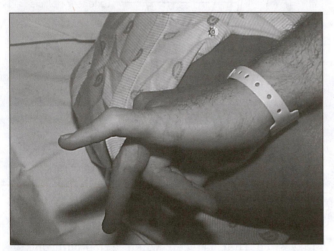

Figure 8-16a. Boutonniere deformity.

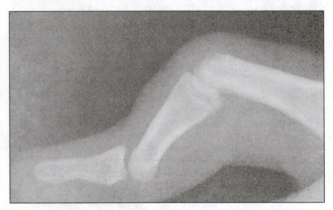

Figure 8-16b. Boutonniere deformity (x-ray).

them, as well as changes in the type of collagen present.[34] Ultimately, this may lead to various deformities of the wrist and hand, loss of range of motion, and decreased strength.

As mentioned, a boutonniere deformity may present itself in the hand as a result of rheumatoid arthritis. In addition, a condition called a swan neck deformity may also develop. This is the outcome of a contracture of the intrinsic muscles. A person with a swan neck deformity will present with flexion of the MP and DIP joints and extension of the PIP joint (Figure 8-17). Both of these conditions can tremendously impact the ability of one to perform activities of daily living and therefore require therapeutic and prophylactic intervention.

OSTEOARTHRITIS

All of the joints in the body are prone to arthritic changes of the joints due to daily wear and tear. Most often, we think of weightbearing joints, such as the knee and hip, as areas that undergo greater amounts of stress. In the wrist

and hand, osteoarthritic changes are often brought about as a result of repetitive and prolonged occupational and recreational habits[35] (Figure 8-18).

To effectively manage osteoarthritis in this area, one must take a close look at the actual task that may be the precursor to these changes. Intervention may include strengthening of the surrounding musculature, modified techniques, and the use of ergonomically designed tools.

Nerve Injuries

Three main peripheral nerves supply motor function and sensation to the wrist and hand area: median, ulnar, and radial. Of these, the median nerve appears to be the most involved from a standpoint of affecting normal function in the hand. This usually occurs in the area referred to as the carpal tunnel. The carpal tunnel is a relatively small section in the hand that contains the median nerve along with the tendons from the flexor digitorum superficialis (4), flexor digitorum profundus

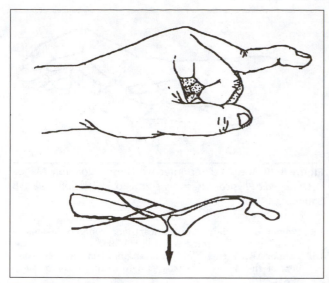

Figure 8-17. Swan neck deformity (reprinted with permission from Magee D. *Orthopedic Physical Assessment*. 2nd ed. Philadelphia, Pa: WB Saunders; 1992).

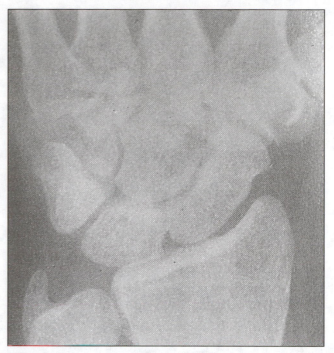

Figure 8-18. Osteoarthritis of wrist.

(4), and flexor pollicis longus (1) muscles. It is bordered on three sides by the carpal bones and on the fourth by the volar carpal ligament[36] (Figure 8-19).

If the median nerve is compressed or altered in any way within this tunnel, both sensory and motor deficits in the hand may be seen upon clinical examination. This can occur from a change in the size of the tunnel, as may be seen with an inflammatory response or a change in the shape of the tunnel's borders as a result of a traumatic incident. This condition is referred to as *carpal tunnel syndrome*. A person may adequately compensate for the symptoms of median nerve injury by the use of vision and the contralateral hand, suggesting that one should closely assess the outcome of performance during daily living tasks through the use of measurement scales.[37,38]

Since the median nerve innervates many of the intrinsic flexor muscles, atrophy of muscle weakness may present upon an assessment of one's grip strength. Eventually, atrophy of the thenar eminence may be pronounced enough to lead to a condition known as *ape hand*[39] (Figure 8-20).

Injury to the ulnar nerve in the wrist and hand area is not as common as it is in the elbow region. However, it may occur, and it too will present itself with a challenge for the clinician who is dealing with a person who has an inability to effectively utilize the interossei muscles for everyday activities. If the condition becomes chronic, both the interossei and medial two lumbricales may be affected and lead to a significant wasting away of the hypothenar musculature. The deformity that presents itself under these circumstances is referred to as *bishop's hand*, secondary to the resemblance of a bishop's gesture[39] (Figure 8-21).

Injuries to the wrist, especially those that are traumatic in nature, may involve the radial nerve. Since the radial nerve primarily innervates the extensor muscles of the wrist, a person who suffers from a palsy or disruption to this nerve is often left with a condition known as *wrist drop*, in which there is an inability to actively extend the wrist.

Injuries to the median, ulnar, or radial nerves must be addressed on a case-by-case basis. The degree of damage to the nerve itself will determine its overall potential to regenerate. Generally speaking, a complete rehabilitation program includes both motor and sensory retraining, as well as the implementation of any adaptations that must be made to accommodate to the injury.[40]

References

1. Norkin C, Levangie P. *Joint Structure and Function: A Comprehensive Analysis*. Philadelphia, Pa: FA Davis; 1983.
2. Soderberg GL. *Kinesiology: Applications to Pathologic Motion*. Baltimore, Md: Williams & Wilkins; 1986.
3. deGroot J. *Correlative Neuroanatomy*. 2nd ed. Norwalk, Conn: Appleton & Lange; 1991.
4. Pratt NE. *Clinical Musculoskeletal Anatomy*. Philadelphia, Pa: JB Lippincott Company; 1991.
5. Warfel JH. *The Extremities: Muscles and Motor Points*. 6th ed. Philadelphia, Pa: Lea & Febiger; 1993.

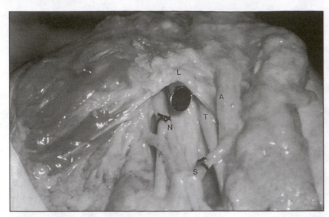

Figure 8-19. Carpal tunnel anatomy.

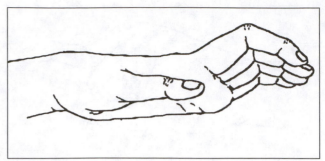

Figure 8-20. Ape hand (reprinted with permission from Magee D. *Orthopedic Physical Assessment.* 2nd ed. Philadelphia, Pa: WB Saunders; 1992).

14. Palmer AK. Triangular fibrocartilage complex lesions: a classification. *J Hand Surg.* 1989; 4:594.
15. Palmer AK, Werner FW. The triangular fibrocartilage complex of the wrist—anatomy and function. *J Hand Surg.* 1981; 2:153.
16. van der Linden AJ. Disk lesions of the wrist joint. *J Hand Surg.* 1986; 4:490.
17. Kapandji IA. *The Physiology of Joints, Vol 1: Upper Limb.* 2nd ed. London: Churchill Livingstone; 1970.
18. Kaplan EB. The participation of the metacarpophalangeal joint of the thumb in the act of opposition. *Bull Hosp Jt Dis.* 1966; 27:39.
19. Lehmkuhl LD, Smith LK. *Brunnstrom's Clinical Kinesiology.* 4th ed. Philadelphia, Pa: FA Davis; 1983.
20. Cooney WP, Chao EYS. Biomechanical analysis of static forces of the thumb during hand function. *J Bone Joint Surg.* 1981; 59:27-36.
21. Napier JR. The prehensile movements of the human hand. *J Bone Joint Surg.* 1956; 38:902.
22. Landsmeer JMF. Power grip and precision handling. *Ann Rheum Dis.* 1962; 22:164.
23. Hamilton GF, McDonald C, Chenier TC. Measurement of grip strength: validity and reliability of the sphygmomanometer and jamar grip dynamometer. *J Orthop Sport Phys Ther.* 1992; 5:215-219.
24. Ketchum LD. A clinical study of the forces generated by the intrinsic muscles of the index finger and extrinsic flexor and extensor muscles of the hand. *J Hand Surg.* 1978; 6:571.
25. Chao EY, Opgrande JD, Axmear FE. Three-dimensional force analysis of finger joints in selected isometric hand functions. *J Biomech.* 1976; 6:387.
26. Harty M. The hand of man. *Phys Ther.* 1974; 7:777.
27. Hazelton FT, Smidt GL, Flatt AE. The influence of wrist position on the force produced by the flexors. *J Biomech.* 1975; 8:301-306.
28. Angermann P, Lohmann M. Injuries to the hand and wrist—a study of 50,272 injuries. *Acta Orthop Scand.* 1994; s262:21.
29. Hackel ME, Wolfe GA, Bang SM, Canfield JS. Changes in hand function in the aging adult as determined by the Jebson test of hand function. *Phys Ther.* 1992; 5:373-377.
30. Canelon MF. Material properties: a factor in the selection and application of splinting materials for athletic wrist and hand injuries. *J Orthop Sport Phys Ther.* 1995; 4:164-172.
31. McCue FC, Mayer V, Moran DJ. Gamekeeper's thumb: ulnar collateral ligament rupture. *J Musculoskeletal Medicine.* 1988; 5:53-63.
32. Gieck JH, Mayer V. Protective splinting for the hand and wrist. *Clin Sports Med.* 1986; 5:795-807.
33. Barden W, Brooks D, Ayling-Campos A. Physical therapy management of the subluxated wrist in children with arthritis. *Phys Ther.* 1995; 10:879-885.

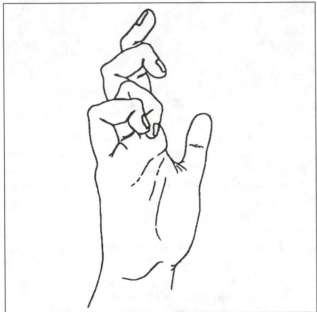

Figure 8-21. Bishop's hand (reprinted with permission from Magee D. *Orthopedic Physical Assessment.* 2nd ed. Philadelphia, Pa: WB Saunders; 1992).

6. Hoppenfeld S. *Physical Examination of the Spine and Extremities.* Norwalk, Conn: Appleton & Lange; 1976.
7. Agur AMR. *Grant's Atlas of Anatomy.* 9th ed. Baltimore, Md: Williams & Wilkins; 1991.
8. Whipple TL. *Arthroscopic Surgery: The Wrist.* Philadelphia, Pa: JB Lippincott Company; 1992.
9. Sennwald CR, Zdrakovic V, Jacob HAC, Kern HP. Kinematic analysis of relative motion within the proximal carpal row. *J Hand Surg.* 1993; 5:609-612.
10. Volz RG, Lieb M, Benjamin J. Biomechanics of the wrist. *Clin Orthop.* 1980; 149:112-117.
11. Sarrafian SK, Melamed JL, Goshgarian GM. Study of wrist motion in flexion and extension. *Clin Orthop.* 1974; 104:92-111.
12. Mayfield JK, Johnson RP, Kilcoyne RF. The ligaments of the human wrist and their functional significance. *Anat Rec.* 1976; 3:417.
13. Youm Y. Kinematics of the wrist, I: an experimental study of radial-ulnar deviation and flexion-extension. *J Bone Joint Surg.* 1978; 3:205.

34. Benjamin M, Ralphs JR, Shibu M, Irwin M. Capsular tissues of the proximal interphalangeal joint: normal composition and effects of dupuytren's disease and rheumatoid arthritis. *J Hand Surg.* 1993;3:371-376.

35. Kisner C, Colby LA. *Therapeutic Exercise: Foundations and Techniques.* 2nd ed. Philadelphia, Pa: FA Davis; 1990.

36. Rasch PJ. *Kinesiology and Applied Anatomy.* 7th ed. Philadelphia, Pa: Lea & Febiger; 1989.

37. Jerosch-Herold C. Measuring outcome in median nerve injuries. *J Hand Surg.* 1993; 5:624-628.

38. Levine DW, Simmons BP, Koris MJ, et al. A self-administered questionnaire for the assessment of severity of symptoms and functional status in carpal tunnel syndrome. *J Bone Joint Surg.* 1993; 11:1585-1592.

39. Magee DJ. *Orthopedic Physical Assessment.* Philadelphia, Pa: WB Saunders; 1992.

40. Wynn-Parry CB. *Rehabilitation of the Hand.* 4th ed. London: Butterworth; 1981.

1. Identify and palpate the carpal bones of the wrist.

2. Demonstrate how active insufficiency of the wrist can affect overall grip strength.

3. Why is it difficult to measure wrist joint range of motion with a goniometer?

4. What positions of the wrist would potentially compromise the integrity of the median nerve?

5. Perform the different methods of a power grip. Explain how different muscles are utilized during each grip type.

6. How would precision handling techniques be affected with a paralysis of the median nerve? Ulnar nerve?

7. How would not having any of the essential requirements for prehensile functions specifically affect one's ability to operate?

8. Passively take each joint of the wrist and hand to its end ranges. What are the stabilizing structures that prevent further movement from occurring?

9. Demonstrate the mechanism of injury for each of the following conditions: a. mallet finger; b. jersey finger; c. boutonniere deformity.

10. List specific activities or occupations that could lead to wrist and hand injuries. Which of these would you classify as overuse injuries? Which might occur as a result of compression? Vibration? Distraction?

11. Explain why grip-like activities may not be beneficial for a person with a carpal ligament tear.

12. Describe the functional position of the hand.

13. Using a partner, label the convex and concave joint articulations of the wrist and hand.

14. Explain how the extrinsic muscles can contribute to movement of multiple joints within the wrist and hand.

CHAPTER 9

SPINE AND POSTURE

Scott Biely, MS, PT

OBJECTIVES

After completion of this chapter, the reader will be able to:

DIDACTIC

1. Explain the functions of the spine as a whole.
2. Describe the functional spinal unit.
3. Explain the role of the intervertebral disc in weightbearing and movement.
4. Identify the different regions and curves of the spine.
5. Compare and contrast the orientation of the facet joints in the different regions of the spine and explain their effect on movement.
6. Identify limiting factors to spinal movement.
7. Explain the role of different muscles in moving and stabilizing the spine.
8. Describe the sacroiliac joint and its role in weightbearing.

PRACTICAL

1. Demonstrate the movements occurring in the spine as a whole.
2. Demonstrate the differences between lower and upper cervical movement.
3. Demonstrate the effect of spinal posture on other areas of the body.

The spine is unique in the functional requirements it must meet. It must be strong and stable to support the trunk and protect the sensitive neural tissue of the spinal cord, but it must also be flexible to allow movement of the head and extremities. Three primary functions are required of the spine:[1]

1. It serves as the central pillar of the trunk. This involves supporting the head and extremities and providing a site of attachment for many of the muscles that stabilize or move the extremities. In addition, this central pillar allows for the transfer of forces through the body and provides some shock absorption of those forces.

2. It forms a protective, bony canal through which the spinal cord and spinal nerve roots pass. This affords the neural tissue some amount of bony protection to the point where the spinal nerves exit from the intervertebral foramina.

3. It provides a wide range of movement, which allows the position of the head and the visual field to be altered and allows the hands and feet to be positioned in space for varying tasks. The mobility of the spine also contributes to locomotion.

THE FUNCTIONAL SPINAL UNIT: THE MOTION SEGMENT

With the exception of the first two vertebrae, each vertebra is separated from the vertebrae above and below it by an intervertebral disc. Panjabi[2] describes the *functional spinal unit* as two adjacent vertebrae and the intervertebral disc that separates them (Figure 9-1) and identifies it as the smallest moveable segment of the spine. This concept of the functional spinal unit or motion segment allows the basic movements of the spine to be identified and studied.

Bony Elements: The Vertebrae

Vertebrae vary considerably in different regions of the spine but possess similar basic elements.[3] Each typical vertebra can be divided into two main sections: the vertebral body and the vertebral or neural arch (Figure 9-2).

The vertebral body is roughly cylindrical in shape. It is convex in the transverse plane except along the posterior aspect, where it is concave.

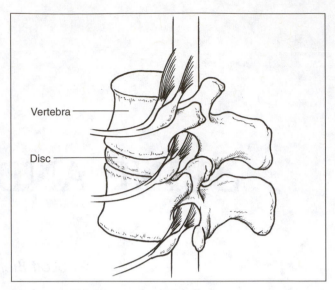

Figure 9-1. The functional spinal unit.

Projecting posteriorly from the vertebral body are two short, broad, bony bars known as the *pedicles*. Another short, broad, bony bar, known as the *lamina* projects posteriorly and medially from each pedicle. The two laminae join in the midline to form a continuous bony ring that consists of the posterior aspect of the vertebral body, the two pedicles, and the two laminae. This ring encircles the vertebral foramen through which the spinal cord passes.

Several processes arise from the junction of the pedicle with the lamina.[3] A transverse process projects laterally from this junction and serves as an attachment point for many of the muscles that move the spine. Articular processes, or zygapophyses, project superiorly and inferiorly from this junction. The superior articular process possesses an articular surface that faces posteriorly and sometimes laterally. The inferior articular process possesses an articular surface that faces anteriorly and sometimes medially.

Each of these three processes is paired with a similar process at the pedicle and lamina junction on the contralateral side of the spine. This creates three paired, or six total, processes. A seventh process, the spinous process, arises in the midline at the junction of the two laminae. The spinous process projects posteriorly and sometimes inferiorly and serves as an attachment site for muscles moving the spine[3] and the extremities.[4]

The superior and inferior surfaces of each vertebral body are flattened to allow for the attachment of the intervertebral disc. Thus, two adjacent vertebral bodies are attached to each other by this

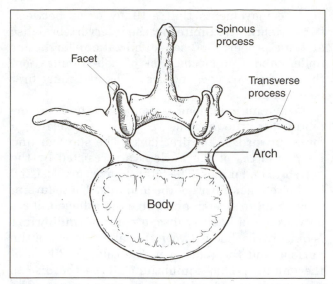

Figure 9-2. Vertebral body and neural arch.

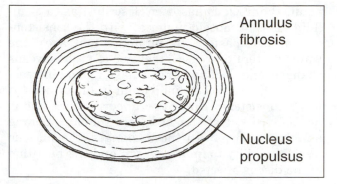

Figure 9-3. Components of the intervertebral disc.

disc.[3] The inferior articular processes of one vertebra articulate with the superior articular processes of the vertebra below it to create the *zygapophyseal* or *facet joints*.[5] The paired facet joints create two additional points of attachment between two vertebrae. The stacking of one vertebra upon another creates a foramen bound by the vertebral bodies, the intervertebral disc, the two pedicles, and the superior and inferior articular processes.[3] This foramen is identified as the *intervertebral foramen*, and through it passes the spinal nerve root. In addition, the stacking of the vertebrae creates a canal from adjacent vertebral foramina. This canal is known as the *vertebral* or *spinal canal* and houses the spinal cord and spinal nerve roots.

The Intervertebral Disc

Movement in the functional spinal unit occurs at the facet joints and the intervertebral disc. The intervertebral disc has two primary functions: it allows movement between vertebral bodies, and it transmits loads from one vertebra to the next.[6] It consists of two primary components: the central nucleus pulposus and the surrounding annulus fibrosus (Figure 9-3).

NUCLEUS PULPOSUS

The nucleus pulposus is located in the central or posterior central portion of the disc. It is composed of water, proteoglycans, collagen fibers, a few cartilage cells, and a small amount of other proteins.[6] By far, the largest component is water. Because of the high water content, the nucleus

obeys the rules of fluid dynamics. It can be deformed under pressure but cannot be compressed. When subjected to pressure, it will deform and transmit the pressure in all directions.[6]

Although the nucleus cannot be compressed when a force is applied to it, a sustained load can gradually force water to leave the nucleus and can decrease the water content of the nucleus.[8] This results in a decrease in the size of the nucleus. The nucleus is separated from the vertebral body by the *vertebral end plates*.[6] These end plates are cartilaginous and are closely attached to the intervertebral disc, except for its outermost layers. The end plates contain microscopic pores that allow water to pass out of and into the nucleus. When a sustained load is applied to the nucleus, water passes from the nucleus, through the vertebral end plates, and into the spongy bone of the vertebral body.

The proteoglycan component of the nucleus has the ability to attract and retain water.[6] Thus, when a load is removed from the nucleus, water passes from the vertebral body back into the nucleus, and the nucleus increases in size. When an individual lies down to sleep, the disc is unloaded, and water enters the nucleus. The nucleus also increases in size while the individual is resting. During an average night of sleep, an individual may gain 2 cm of height because of an increase in the size of the nuclei.[8] In space travel, astronauts are not subjected to the compressive forces of gravity and may gain 5 to 10 cm of height.[7] When the individual assumes an upright posture, the disc is loaded, and water is forced back out of the disc. The nucleus decreases in size, and the individual loses height.[8]

The regular loading and unloading of the disc and dehydration and hydration of the nucleus are important in the nutrition of the disc.[5] A disturbance of these cycles may affect the nutrition and health of the nucleus. The components of the nucleus vary considerably with age. In a healthy young adult, the nucleus has been described as "a semi-fluid mass of mucoid material with the consistency... of toothpaste."[6] As an individual ages, the water content decreases, the type of proteoglycans changes, and the number of collagen fibers increases.[5] The nucleus of an individual in his or her 40s has a consistency closer to cranberry sauce and is not as easily distinguished from the surrounding annulus.[9] Along with these changes, the nucleus loses its ability to imbibe water, and the nutrition of the disc is affected.

ANNULUS FIBROSUS

The annulus fibrosus consists of concentric rings of obliquely oriented collagen fibers. The fibers in each layer, or lamella, are parallel to each other but angled 65° to 70° from the vertical.[6] The direction of the fibers alternates with each successive lamellae. Thus, in one lamellae the collagen fibers are angled 65° to the right of the vertical, but in the next layer the fibers are oriented 65° to the left of the vertical. These lamellae are thick anteriorly and laterally but are thinner and more tightly packed posteriorly.

The fibers and lamellae are tightly bound to each other by a proteoglycan gel.[6] The proteoglycans in the annulus are also capable of attracting and retaining water, which is also the principal component of the annulus. In addition, the annulus contains cartilage cells and elastin fibers.

The nucleus and the annulus are very similar biochemically.[6] They differ only in the percentage of different components and in the type of collagen fibers. In reality, the boundary between the inner annulus and the outer nucleus is very difficult to discern.

Mechanics of Movement

The nucleus encased within the annulus is roughly spherical in shape. Because it is primarily fluid, it cannot be compressed. Thus, the nucleus acts like a ball placed between two planes, and the movements between two adjacent vertebrae can be likened to a swivel joint.[8] In this sense, the intervertebral articulation possesses 6° of freedom and allows the following motions: tilting forward and backward in the sagittal plane (flexion and extension), gliding in the sagittal plane (anterior and posterior shear), tilting in the frontal plane (right and left lateral flexion), gliding in the frontal plane (right and left lateral shear), rotation in the transverse plane (right and left rotation), and gliding along the longitudinal axis (distraction and compression).[7,8]

The movements that actually occur between two vertebrae are limited by the intervertebral disc and its property of self-stabilization. To better understand the mechanism of self-stabilization, the weightbearing capacities of the disc must first be examined.

When an axial load is applied to the intervertebral disc, the nucleus responds by exerting a force outward in all directions.[5] The superior and inferior forces of the nucleus are resisted by the vertebral end plates. The lateral forces are resisted by the collagen fibers of the annulus. These lateral forces tend to stretch and bulge the collagen fibers outward. In a healthy disc, a point of equilibrium is quickly reached between the lateral forces of the nucleus and the tension in the collagen fibers of the annulus. This equilibrium allows the disc to withstand considerable compressive forces. The fibers of the annulus are braced by pressure from the nucleus, and the load can be passed from one vertebra to the next. In addition, the transfer of the force from the nucleus into the collagen fibers has a shock-absorbing effect.[5]

The oblique orientation of the annulus fibers of the disc limit the movements of distraction, tilting, gliding, and rotation. However, the interaction of the annulus and nucleus provides additional movement constraints.[8] When a vertebra tilts anteriorly, the posterior fibers of the annulus are stretched. However, pressure of the nucleus against those fibers limits the distance those fibers can be stretched and tends to restore the vertebra to its original position. This is the self-stabilization action of the disc.[8]

Because of the ability of the nucleus to imbibe water, the nucleus always maintains a certain amount of pressure against the fibers of the annulus. However, contraction of the spinal muscles often involves a component of compression of the intervertebral discs. The increased compression increases the pressure of the nucleus and further enhances the self-stabilization action.

The Facet Joints

In addition to the intervertebral disc, movement in the functional spinal unit occurs at the facet joints.[5] The paired facet joints are formed by the articulation of the two inferior articular processes of one vertebra with the two superior articular processes of the vertebra below it. The facet joints are synovial joints with hyaline cartilage covering the articular surfaces. The articular surfaces vary throughout the spine from planar in

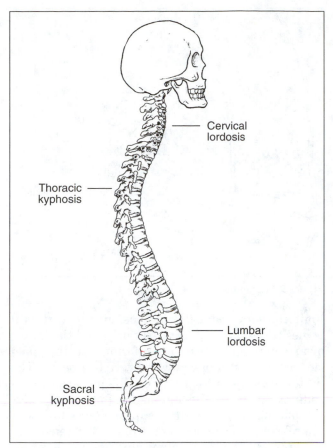

Cervical
lordosis

Thoracic
kyphosis

Lumbar
lordosis

Sacral
kyphosis

Figure 9-4. Anatomical curves of the spine.

the cervical region to convex-concave in the lumbar region with the inferior articular process forming the convex partner and the superior articular process forming the concave partner.[3] In most cases, intervertebral movement involves a sliding of the inferior articular surface on the superior articular surface.

Orientation of the articular surfaces can also vary considerably throughout the spine. This orientation serves to govern the direction and nature of the intervertebral movement.[7] Although the intervertebral articulation possesses 6° of freedom, the orientation of the facet joints allows more movement in certain planes and less in others and limits the degrees of freedom.

The available movement in the different regions of the spine is affected by the surfaces of the facet joints, the orientation of the facet joints, and the proportion of the disc height to the vertebral body height. This will be discussed later in the chapter.

THE SPINE AS A WHOLE

The functional spinal unit provides a useful model for studying segmental movement of the spine, but movement of the spine in the body is affected by many factors that are not included in the functional spinal unit. The 24 vertebrae of the spine and their interposing intervertebral discs form the *vertebral* or *spinal column*. The five fused sacral vertebrae and the three to five fused vertebrae that compose the coccyx are sometimes included as part of the column. Thus, the spinal column can be considered to consist of 26 mobile segments.[10]

The spinal column can be divided into five regions: seven cervical vertebrae; 12 thoracic vertebrae from which the ribs arise; five lumbar vertebrae; five fused vertebrae that form the sacrum, which articulates with the inominate bones of the pelvis; and three to five fused vertebrae that form the coccyx. In the frontal plane, the spinal column appears to be straight. However, in the sagittal plane, four distinct curves can be identified: the cervical lordosis (concave posteriorly), the thoracic kyphosis (convex posteriorly), the lumbar lordosis (concave posteriorly), and the sacral or pelvic curve (convex posteriorly)[8] (Figure 9-4). These curves increase the spinal column's resistance to axial compression. Engineers have shown that the resistance of a curved column to axial compression increases with the number of curves in the column.[8]

The structure of the spinal column is maintained in part by ligaments that run the length of the spine[3] (Figure 9-5). The anterior longitudinal ligament is a broad, flat ligament that runs from the occiput to the sacrum. It attaches to the anterior surface of the intervertebral discs and to the anterior margins of the vertebral bodies. The posterior longitudinal ligament runs from the body of the second cervical vertebra to the sacrum. It attaches to the posterior aspect of the intervertebral discs and to the posterior margins of the vertebral bodies; hence, it lies within the vertebral canal. This ligament is fairly uniform in width in the cervical spine, but in the lumbar spine it is thin over the vertebral bodies and broad over the intervertebral discs. The ligamenta flava also lie within the vertebral canal. They run from the articular capsule of the facet joint and the lamina of one vertebra to the articular capsule and lamina of the vertebra above. The ligamentum flavum is named the "yellow ligament" because of a predominance of yellow elastin fibers.

The interspinous ligaments are thin ligaments that connect the spinous process of one vertebra with the spinous processes of the vertebrae above and below it. These ligaments approach the ligamenta flava anteriorly and the supraspinous ligament posteriorly. The supraspinous ligament is a strong, fibrous ligament that essentially connects the spinous processes of all vertebrae. In the cervical spine, the supraspinous ligament is expanded to form the ligamentum nuchae, which serves as an attachment site for muscles of the neck. The supraspinous ligament then runs from the spinous process of the seventh cervical vertebra to the sacrum.[3]

Movements of the Spine

Although the intervertebral articulation has 6° of freedom, the ligaments and facet joints limit the movement that can occur between vertebrae. As a whole, the spinal column functions as a joint with 3° of freedom.[8] The movements that can be observed clinically include flexion and extension, right and left lateral flexion, and right and left rotation. Strictly defined, flexion involves "bending of a joint to approximate the parts it connects," and extension involves "bringing the distal portion of a joint in continuity with the long axis of the proximal part."[11] In this sense, the initial forward bending of a lordotic segment of the spine is actually extension because the vertebrae are moving toward the long axis of the proximal part. Forward bending of the spine involves extension of the cervical spine, flexion of the thoracic spine, and extension of the lumbar spine.[9] However, for simplicity, flexion refers to forward bending of the spine or moving the spine so the concavity is anterior, and extension refers to backward bending of the spine or moving the spine so the concavity is posterior.[11]

In flexion, the vertebral bodies tilt anteriorly, and the inferior articular processes glide superiorly on the superior articular processes of the vertebra below.[3] The vertebral bodies not only tilt anteriorly but also translate anteriorly.[7] The anterior longitudinal ligament is relaxed, and the anterior annulus is compressed. The movement is limited by tension in the posterior fibers of the annulus, the posterior longitudinal ligament, the interspinous ligament, and the supraspinous ligament. In addition, the elasticity of the ligamenta flava and the tension in the extensor muscles tend to

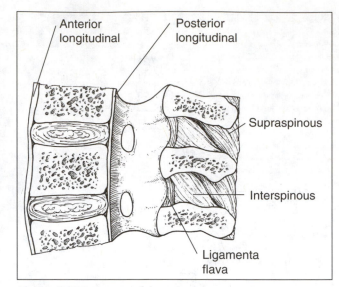

Figure 9-5. Ligaments of the spine.

limit the movement.[3] In extension, the vertebral bodies tilt and translate posteriorly, and the inferior articular processes glide inferiorly on the superior articular processes of the vertebra below. The posterior fibers of the annulus, the posterior longitudinal ligament, the ligamenta flava, the interspinous ligament, and the supraspinous ligament are relaxed. This movement is limited by tension in the anterior fibers of the annulus and the anterior longitudinal ligament. It is also limited by approximation of the spinous processes.[3]

The range of motion of each intervertebral joint may be quite small, but when the movements occurring at each segment are combined, the resultant range of motion can be quite large. Kapandji[8] notes that total ranges vary considerably from one individual to another, especially in individuals of different ages, but he has measured 110° of flexion and 140° of extension or a total of 250° of spinal range of motion in the sagittal plane.

Flexion and extension may be the only spinal movements that occur primarily in one plane. Grieve[7] notes that in lateral flexion and rotation movements, "after the first degree or two of motion, one induces a portion of the other, and they are inseparable." Brunnstrom[12] explains this coupling of motion with a mechanical principle that states, "If a flexible rod is bent first in one plane, and then while it is in this bent position, it is bent again in a plane at right angles to the first, it always rotates on its longitudinal axis at the same time." The normal curves of the spinal column create the first "bend," and a lateral flexion movement would create the second "bend." Thus, the spine

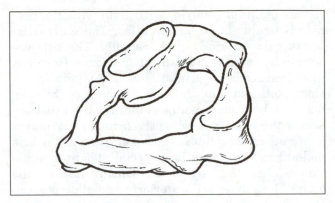

Figure 9-6. First cervical vertebra.

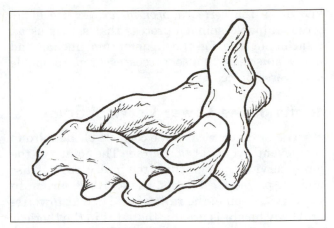

Figure 9-7. Second cervical vertebra.

would rotate in conjunction with a lateral flexion movement. Kapandji[8] feels that the coupling of movement, or "automatic rotation," is caused by compression of the intervertebral discs and stretching of ligaments. Bogduk and Twomey[6] report that the exact mechanism of the coupling has not yet been determined but note that the process probably involves the movement and compression of the facet joints, the torsional and shear stresses on the intervertebral disc, the force of gravity, the direction of the force of muscle contraction, and the shape and position of the natural curves of the spine. Some disagreement exists concerning the direction of the coupled movements. Grieve[7] states that rotation and lateral flexion occur to the same side in the flexed, neutral, or extended cervical spine and in the flexed thoracic and lumbar spine. Rotation and lateral flexion occur to the opposite side in the neutral or extended thoracic and lumbar spine. Bogduk and Twomey[6] note that the pattern and degree of coupling may vary from one individual to another and from one segment to another.

Lateral flexion and rotation are limited by tension in the fibers of the annulus, the surrounding ligaments, and the antagonist muscles. Approximation of the facet joints can also limit rotation.[3] Kapandji[8] has measured 75° of lateral flexion and 90° of rotation of the spinal column.

CERVICAL SPINE

The first two cervical vertebrae vary considerably from the typical vertebrae described earlier. The first cervical vertebra, or C1, is also known as the *atlas* because it supports the "globe" of the head.[3] It is somewhat ring-shaped with two lateral masses, a short anterior arch, and a longer, curved posterior arch (Figure 9-6). The superior surface of

each lateral mass contains a concave surface that articulates with the corresponding convex occipital condyle of the skull. The inferior surface of each lateral mass contains a flat or slightly convex surface that articulates with a similar surface on the second cervical vertebra. The atlas is unique in that it possesses no vertebral body and no true spinous process. The normal position of the vertebral body is occupied by a superior projection from the second cervical vertebra. It also has unusually long, palpable transverse processes that serve as attachment sites for muscles that rotate the head.

The second cervical vertebra, or C2, is also known as the *axis* (Figure 9-7) and serves as a pivot on which the atlas and the head can rotate.[3] A bony projection, the odontoid process or dens, rises superiorly from the vertebral body of the axis and articulates with the posterior aspect of the anterior arch of the atlas. It is held in place by the transverse ligament of the atlas. On each side of the dens, on the superior aspect of the vertebral body and pedicles, are oval surfaces that articulate with the atlas. The axis possesses a large, palpable spinous process that serves as an attachment site for muscles that extend and rotate the head.

The typical cervical vertebrae include C3 through C6.[3] They can be distinguished from vertebrae in other portions of the spine by the presence of a foramen in the transverse process, anterior and posterior tubercles that transform the transverse process into a gutter, and a bifid spinous process. Also, unique to the cervical vertebra are two bony projections that arise from the lateral aspect of the superior surface of the vertebral body. These processes articulate with surfaces on the inferior aspect of the vertebra above and form the joints of Luschka or the uncovertebral joints.

The seventh cervical vertebra, or C7, is also

known as the *vertebra prominens* because of its large, palpable spinous process that serves as an attachment site for the ligamentum nuchae and many muscles.[3] It also possesses large, palpable transverse processes.

Joints of the Lower Cervical Spine

The lower cervical spine consists of the third to the seventh cervical vertebrae. The joints of the lower cervical spine include the intervertebral disc and the paired facet joints, as described earlier. In the cervical spine, the ratio of disc height to vertebral body height is greater than it is in the thoracic spine. This imparts a greater mobility in the intervertebral discs of the cervical spine.[7] The cervical vertebrae are capable of more tilting and more translation than in the thoracic spine.

The facet joints guide and limit movement. In the cervical spine, the facet joints are angled 30° to 60° anterior to the long axis of the spine.[1] The orientation of the facet joints allows flexion and extension, as well as a combination of lateral flexion and rotation to the same side to occur in the intervertebral joints of the C3 through C7. The facet joint capsules are quite lax so that considerable tilting and gliding of the vertebrae can occur.

Unique to the cervical spine are the paired uncovertebral joints. The intervertebral disc does not extend to the lateral margins of the cervical vertebral body. Instead, the lateral margins of the vertebral body are raised to form two bony projections. These projections, or uniform processes, contain articular surfaces that face superiorly and medially. They join articular surfaces on the inferior surface of the vertebra above to form the uncovertebral or cervical interbody joints.[13] The articular capsule of these joints is continuous with the outer layers of the annulus. The uncovertebral joints have recently been identified as saddle joints[14]—they allow flexion and extension in the sagittal plane and an axial rotation in the plane of the facet joint. Clefts form in the posterior annulus to allow the posterior half of the vertebral body to rotate in the plane of the facet joint. If the annulus was intact, the axial rotation could not occur.[14] The uncovertebral joints also limit lateral shear.[13]

Joints of the Upper Cervical Spine

The upper cervical spine contains the specialized atlanto-occipital and atlanto-axial joints. The atlanto-occipital joint exists between the occipital condyles of the skull and the atlas (or C1).[3] The convex occipital condyles articulate with the concave articular facets of the atlas. These articular facets run anteriorly and medially. The atlanto-occipital joint possesses 3° of freedom.[8] However, movement consists primarily of flexion and extension. Rotation and lateral flexion are blocked because these movements would involve a distraction of the joint.[14] Because the primary movement occurring at this joint is flexion and extension, or a nodding motion, the atlanto-occipital joint is sometimes called the "yes" joint. During flexion, the occipital condyles roll anteriorly and glide posteriorly. The opposite occurs with extension.

The atlanto-axial joint is actually a complex of three joints.[8] The central joint consists of the articulation of the odontoid process with the anterior arch of the atlas and the transverse ligament, and the two lateral joints consist of the articulation between the superior facets of the axis and the inferior facets of the atlas. The atlanto-axial joint possesses 3° of freedom and allows rotation, lateral flexion, and flexion and extension.[8] However, the primary movement occurring at this joint is rotation. Because rotation is the primary movement, the atlanto-axial joint is sometimes called the "no" joint. During rotation, the head and atlas rotate about the odontoid process. The atlas moves anteriorly on one side and posteriorly on the opposite side. During flexion and extension, the atlas rolls and glides on the axis at the lateral joints. The transverse ligament keeps the odontoid process in contact with the anterior arch of the atlas.[8] The atlas is not bound directly to the axis by any strong ligaments and has few muscle attachments. This allows the atlas to function as a washer between the skull and the axis.[14] It also allows the movements of the atlas to be quite variable depending on the position of the head on the atlas.

The upper cervical spine is supported by a complex of ligaments that provide some stability while still permitting considerable mobility.[13] The alar and apical ligaments attach the odontoid process to the occiput. The position of the odontoid is further reinforced by the cruciate ligament complex. This complex consists of a transverse ligament that runs from one side of the atlas to the other posterior to the odontoid process, an ascending band that attaches to the occiput and a descending band that attaches to the axis. Other ligaments that support this area are continuations of ligaments from the lower cervical spine. The anterior longitudinal ligament becomes the atlanto-occipital membrane attaching to the atlas, axis, and occiput. The posterior longitudinal ligament becomes the tectorial

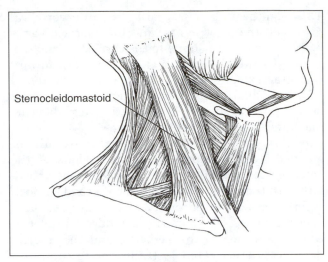

Figure 9-8. Sternocleidomastoid muscle.

membrane and also attaches to the atlas, axis, and occiput. Comparable to the ligamenta flava are the posterior atlanto-occipital and posterior atlanto-axial membranes.[13]

Movements of the Cervical Spine

The gross movements of flexion and extension, rotation, and lateral flexion actually involve combinations of movements from the different joints of the cervical spine. For example, flexion involves anterior tilting and anterior translation of the vertebral bodies as allowed by the intervertebral discs and the uncovertebral joints, anterior and superior glide of the inferior articular processes on the superior articular processes of the facet joints, anterior rolling of the atlas on the axis, and anterior rolling and posterior gliding of the occipital condyles on the atlas. In extension, the opposite movements occur.

The final position of the head in certain movements requires adjustments from the atlanto-axial and atlanto-occipital joints of the upper cervical spine.[9] The gross movement of rotation to the right involves right lateral flexion and rotation of the lower cervical spine. The final position of the head with the chin over the shoulder requires additional right rotation at the atlanto-axial joint and extension at the atlanto-occipital joint. The gross movement of lateral flexion to the right also involves right lateral flexion and rotation of the lower cervical spine. However, to position the head with the face looking forward, the atlanto-axial joint must rotate to the left and the atlanto-occipital joint must extend. Final positioning of the head is largely the responsibility of the upper cervical spine.[9,13]

The cervical spine is more mobile than the other portions of the spine and is designed to meet the requirements of positioning the head in space and altering the visual field. Many studies have investigated the quantity of movement that occurs in the cervical spine.[7,15-18] Recent studies have revealed 140° of movement in the sagittal plane (flexion and extension), 153° of movement in the transverse plane (rotation), and 91° of movement in the frontal plane (lateral flexion).[8]

Muscle Function

Anteriorly, the rectus capitis anterior and rectus capitis lateralis, and posteriorly, the rectus capitis posterior major and minor and the obliquus capitis superior and inferior function to move the head and the upper cervical spine independently of the lower cervical spine.[13]

Moving posteriorly from the suboccipital muscles, the next muscle group is the semispinalis capitis and cervicis, which are important extensors of the head and cervical spine. Posterior to the semispinalis is the trapezius. The trapezius adds stability to the head and neck in the frontal plane. Moving laterally from the suboccipital muscles, the next group is the longissimus capitis and cervicis, which laterally flex the head and cervical spine and provide frontal plane stability. Lateral to the longissimus is the splenius capitis and cervicis, which extend and rotate the head and neck. Lateral to the splenius is the sternocleidomastoid. The sternocleidomastoid has numerous actions, including rotation of the head and neck, extension of the upper cervical spine, and flexion of the lower cervical spine. It also acts to limit extension and posterior translation. This mechanism often causes damage to this muscle in whiplash injuries. Working with the trapezius, it adds stability in the sagittal plane (Figure 9-8).[13]

The scalene muscles laterally flex the neck and provide frontal plane stability. Working with the levator scapulae, they also add stability in the sagittal plane.[13]

The anterior muscles of the neck include the longus colli and capitis, which function as flexors of the cervical spine. The infra- and suprahyoid muscles are the most superficial muscles of the anterior neck and are important in neck posture as well as swallowing, chewing, and talking.[13] Additional information about the muscles of the cervical spine can be found in Appendix A.

Clinical Applications

FORWARD HEAD POSTURE

One of the most common problems seen in patients with neck pain is the presence of a forward head posture. This posture places the head in front of the line of gravity and involves an increase in the thoracic kyphosis in the upper thoracic spine, an increase in the cervical lordosis in the mid cervical spine, and extension at the atlanto-occipital joint. This posture can create a multitude of problems, including the following:

1. Suboccipital headaches caused by pinching of the greater occipital nerve in a narrowed suboccipital space.
2. Temperomandibular joint (TMJ) dysfunction caused by altering the occlusal relationship of the teeth.
3. Loss of upper thoracic mobility secondary to an increased thoracic kyphosis.
4. Increase in lower cervical mobility with resultant degenerative changes in the intervertebral discs.
5. Thoracic outlet problems secondary to tightening of the anterior cervical and chest musculature.
6. Diminished respiratory capacity secondary to decreased ability to use the diaphragm in breathing.
7. Loss of shoulder range of motion secondary to changes in scapular position.

ADVERSE NEURAL TENSION

As the spinal column changes its position, the contained neural tissue must adapt to this movement.[19] The spinal canal is 5 to 9 cm longer in flexion than it is in extension. The bed of the median nerve increases in length by 20% as the wrist and elbow move from flexion to extension. Thus, the neural tissue must be able to move and elongate. Injury to the neck may limit this ability. Thus, tension can develop in the neural tissue, and the health of the tissue may be in jeopardy. This can lead to neurological symptoms at other points in the nervous system. A neck injury may increase an individual's susceptibility to carpal tunnel syndrome.[19]

THORACIC SPINE

The upper portion of the thoracic spine functions very similarly to the cervical spine.[9] Above T3, weightbearing is shared by the intervertebral discs and the facet joints, and the thoracic vertebrae are similar in shape to the cervical vertebrae. Below T3, weightbearing is shifted more toward the intervertebral discs. The size of the vertebral bodies gradually increases through the remainder of the thoracic spine.[3] This shift in weightbearing may affect the pattern of coupling.[6]

The typical thoracic vertebrae are distinguished from vertebrae in other regions of the spine by the presence of costal facets that articulate with the head of the ribs.[3] The second through eighth thoracic vertebrae, T2 to T8, have two pairs of costal facets. The superior demifacets are located just anterior to the pedicles, and the inferior demifacets are located just anterior to the intervertebral foramina. The inferior demifacet of one vertebra and the superior demifacet of the vertebra below form an articular surface that joins with the head of the rib. The rib number corresponds to the number of the thoracic vertebra that contributes the superior demifacet to the articulation. The transverse process of each typical thoracic vertebra possesses a facet that articulates with the tubercle of the corresponding rib. The spinous processes slant inferiorly and posteriorly.

The first thoracic vertebra, or T1, differs from the other thoracic vertebrae in that its superior costal facet is a complete facet instead of a demifacet.[3] It articulates with the head of the first rib. The 10th through 12th thoracic vertebrae, T10 to T12, also have complete superior costal facets. Their vertebral bodies contain no inferior costal facets.[3] The transverse processes of T11 and T12 possess no articular facets.

Joints of the Thoracic Spine

The joints of the thoracic spine include not only the intervertebral disc and paired facet joints, but also the costovertebral and costotransverse joints that attach the ribs to the thoracic spine. In the thoracic spine, the ratio of disc height to vertebral body height is much less than it is in the other regions of the spine.[7] This limits the mobility of the thoracic spine.

The facet joints consist of a flat or slightly convex superior articular process that faces posteriorly, slightly superiorly, and slightly laterally, and a flat or slightly concave inferior articular process that faces anteriorly, slightly inferiorly, and slightly medially.[3] The orientation of the facet allows flexion and extension and a combination of lateral flexion and rotation.

The movements of the thoracic spine are largely affected by the presence and attachments of the ribs. The costovertebral joint is a synovial joint consisting of a concave costal facet formed in most cases by the superior demifacet of one vertebra, a portion of the annulus fibrosus, and the inferior demifacet of the vertebra above.[8] The costal facet articulates with the convex head of the rib. The position of the rib is supported by an interosseous ligament that attaches the rib to the intervertebral disc and a radiate ligament that attaches the rib to the adjacent vertebral bodies and the intervertebral disc.[8]

The costotransverse joint consists of an articular facet on the tip of the transverse process and another on the costal tubercle.[3] The position of the rib is further supported by an interosseous costotransverse ligament that attaches the neck of the rib to the transverse process, a posterior costotransverse ligament that attaches the tip of the transverse process to the costal tubercle, and a superior costotransverse ligament that attaches the transverse process to the neck of the underlying rib.[8]

Movements of the Thoracic Spine

During flexion of the thoracic spine, the inferior articular processes glide superiorly and anteriorly on the superior articular processes. The anterior tilting of the vertebral body is accompanied by some anterior translation. The nearly vertical orientation of the thoracic facet joints limits the amount of flexion.[3] Flexion is also limited by the approximation of the ribs anteriorly and tension in the posterior ligaments. During extension, the vertebral body tilts and translates posteriorly. Extension is limited by the approximation of the articular processes and the spinous processes.[3]

The orientation of the thoracic facet joints would allow considerable lateral flexion. The inferior articular process on one side glides superiorly while the contralateral inferior articular process glides inferiorly. However, approximation of the articular processes and approximation of the ribs on the ipsilateral side limit the lateral flexion.[3]

Lateral flexion is accompanied by rotation, although the direction and amount of the rotation can vary.[20] Rotation results in a distortion of the corresponding rib pair which also limits the total movement.[8]

LUMBAR SPINE

The lumbar vertebrae are distinguished from vertebrae in other regions of the spine by their larger vertebral bodies and short, stout spinous processes.[3] The larger vertebral bodies increase the weightbearing capacity of the lumbar spine.

Joints of the Lumbar Spine

The joints of the lumbar spine include the intervertebral discs and the facet joints. The ratio of disc height to vertebral body height is larger in the lumbar spine than in any other region. This should allow considerable movement.[7]

The facet joints consist of a concave, vertical superior articular process that faces posteriorly and medially and a convex, vertical inferior articular process that faces anteriorly and laterally.[3] The orientation of the facet joints allows considerable movement in the sagittal plane and less movement in the frontal and transverse planes. Thus, flexion and extension predominate, but some lateral flexion and rotation is allowed.[3,7,8] Rotation is limited by compression within the contralateral facet joint.

Whereas the construction of the cervical spine lends to its mobility, the construction of the lumbar spine is more suited to stability. Adding to the stability in the lumbar spine is the presence of the iliolumbar ligament.[21] The iliolumbar ligament runs from the transverse process of the fifth lumbar vertebra (L5), and sometimes the fourth (L4), to the sacrum and iliac crest and serves to anchor L5 to the sacrum[3] (Figure 9-9). It limits movement in the frontal plane and prevents anterior shear.[5]

Movements of the Lumbar Spine

Flexion of the lumbar spine involves anterior tilting and anterior translation of the vertebral body as in the cervical and thoracic spine. Extension involves the opposite movements.[3] Some rotation and lateral flexion can occur, but it is quite limited.[22] The normal center of rotation in the lumbar spine is in the posterior aspect of the intervertebral disc. However, attempting to rotate a lumbar vertebra past its normal range causes compression of the contralateral facet joint[23] and shifts the center of rotation toward the compressed facet.[24] Further movement about this new center of rotation places extreme shear forces on the disc and may lead to damage of the disc.[5,25]

Many studies have investigated the amount of movement in the lumbar spine.[7,8,26] These amounts decrease considerably as a person ages. Studies have measured as much as 60° of flexion, 35° of extension, and 28° of lateral flexion.[7] Measurements of rotation vary from 23° to 5°.[7,8]

Muscle Function

The muscles of the back can be divided into three layers:[3] the superficial layer includes the trapezius, latissimus dorsi, rhomboids, and levator scapulae. These muscles are located on the back but are functionally related to the upper extremities. The intermediate layer includes the serratus posterior superior and inferior. These muscles are functionally related to respiration. The deep layer includes the true back muscles.

The deep layer of back muscles can also be divided into three groups: the first group is the longitudinal muscles, which are also known as the erector spinae or the sacrospinalis. This group includes the iliocostalis, the longissimus, and the spinalis. These muscles extend the spine and act unilaterally to contribute to lateral flexion. The second group is the oblique or transversospinal muscles and includes the semispinalis, multifidus, and rotatores longus and brevis. These muscles function in rotation and acting bilaterally to contribute to extension. The third group is the segmental muscles, which include the interspinales and intertransversari. These muscles contain such a small cross-sectional area that they are probably more important in proprioception than they are in movement.[28]

The flexors of the spine are the abdominal muscles, which are positioned anterior to the axis of movement. These muscles include the external and internal oblique, the transversus abdominis, and the rectus abdominis. The oblique abdominal muscles also participate in rotation.[5] Please refer to Appendix A for further information on these muscles.

The importance of stability in the lumbar spine is further emphasized by the function of the muscles that attach to the lumbar spine.[5] The lumbar spine is surrounded by a group of muscles that serve as core stabilizers of the lumbar spine in all planes. The deep portions of the iliocostalis lumborum and the longissimus thoracis are prime extensors of the lumbar spine but also serve to limit flex-

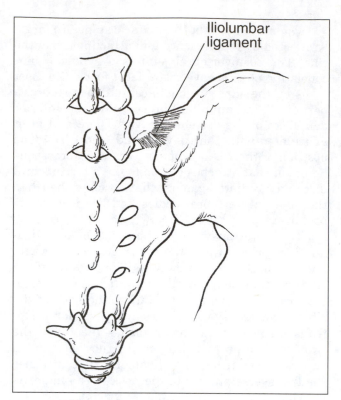

Figure 9-9. The iliolumbar ligament.

ion and anterior shear.[29] The multifidus is optimally positioned to aid in this function. In addition, the multifidus has been shown to possess a greater number of type I fibers and probably has more of a postural or stabilizing function.[5] The position of the psoas muscle allows it to counterbalance the functions of the multifidus and the deep portions of the iliocostalis lumborum and longissimus thoracis. It resists extension and posterior shear. The psoas has been shown to be more active than many trunk muscles in different positions.[5] These muscles create sagittal plane stability for the lumbar spine. The quadratus lumborum provides stability in the frontal plane and limits lateral flexion.[5] No extensor muscle of the lumbar spine possesses a long enough lever arm to provide stability in the transverse plane and limit rotation. However, the internal oblique and transversus abdominis attach to the transverse processes of the lumbar spine through the thoracolumbar fascia and can function as anti-rotation muscles.[5] Thus, stability of the lumbar spine is achieved in all planes.

In addition to moving and stabilizing the lumbar spine, most muscles provide a compressive force through the lumbar spine. This compressive force is resisted by the expansion of the nucleus pulposus and increases the tension in the fibers of

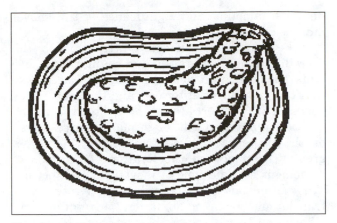

Figure 9-10. Damage to the annulus.

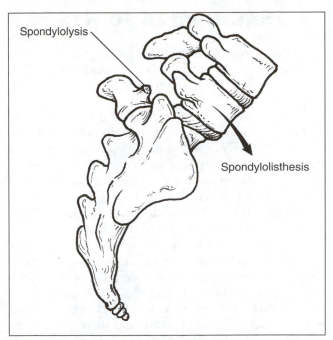

Figure 9-11. Spondylolysis and spondylolisthesis.

the annulus fibrosus. Thus, further stability is achieved by limiting the amount of movement allowed by the intervertebral disc.[5]

One additional source of stability is the thoracolumbar fascia, which has been likened to a tent supported underneath by the erector spinae muscles, the multifidus, and the quadratus lumborum and attached on the sides by the latissimus dorsi, gluteus maximus, transversus abdominis, and internal oblique muscles.[5] Contraction of these muscles tightens the fabric of the tent and adds stability to the trunk.

Clinical Applications

THE "SLIPPED DISC" OR HERNIATED NUCLEUS PULPOSUS

The posterior aspect of the annulus fibrosus is subject to compression, torsion, bending, and shear forces and is vulnerable to injury. This damage to the annulus is the beginning of disc pathology.[5] The annulus loses its effectiveness at limiting vertebral movement and containing the nucleus.[30] The initial annular damage may be caused by an isolated trauma such as a fall or motor vehicle accident, or by the accumulation of smaller stresses caused by daily activities. As damage to the annulus accumulates, the nucleus may eventually move through cracks and tears in the annulus[5] (Figure 9-10). Positions that increase nucleus pressure facilitate this movement. The end result is a herniation of nuclear material through the annulus.

SPONDYLOLYSIS

The lordotic curve of the lumbar spine and the anterior tilting of the sacrum place the lower lumbar vertebrae on an incline. The forces of gravity accentuated by any compressive load on the spine create a resultant force that tends to slide the vertebral bodies of the lower lumbar vertebrae inferiorly and anteriorly down this incline.[8] This anterior sliding is resisted by the wedging of the inferior articular processes against the superior articular processes of the vertebra below. These forces create a stress in the pars interarticularis or vertebral isthmus, a portion of bone that lies between the inferior and superior articular processes. Excessive compressive or extension forces may lead to fracture of the pars interarticularis, a condition known as spondylolysis. The vertebral body is no longer restrained by the articular processes and may now slip inferiorly and anteriorly. This resultant anterior translation is known as spondylolisthesis. The conditions of spondylolysis and spondylolisthesis are visible in oblique x-rays of the lumbar spine. An oblique view of the lumbar spine creates an image of a "Scotty dog," in which the transverse process is the head of the dog, the lamina is the body, the inferior articular process is the front leg, the spinous process is the rear leg, and the superior articular process is the ear. In spondylolysis, the Scotty dog will appear to be wearing a collar. In spondylolisthesis, the Scotty dog will appear to be decapitated[8] (Figure 9-11).

SACROILIAC JOINTS

The sacroiliac joints attach the sacrum to the iliac bones of the pelvis and serve as a connection between the axial skeleton and the lower extremities.

The sacrum is a wedge-shaped mass of bone formed by fusion of the five sacral vertebrae.[3] It is wider superiorly and anteriorly than inferiorly and posteriorly. The superior surface of the sacrum is known as the base. It is actually the superior surface of S1 and attaches to the fifth lumbar vertebra through an intervertebral disc and two paired facet joints. The inferior surface of the sacrum is known as the apex. It is the inferior surface of S5 and articulates with the coccyx. The lateral aspect of the sacrum possesses an ear-shaped articular surface known as the auricular surface. The auricular surface has a shorter, nearly vertical, cephalic limb over the lateral aspect of S1 and a longer, nearly horizontal, caudal limb that extends over the lateral aspect of S2 and S3.[3]

The ilium contains a similarly shaped auricular surface that articulates with the sacrum.[3] The ilium is fused with the ischium and pubis bones to form an inominate bone. The paired inominate bones and sacrum together form the pelvis. In addition to the sacroiliac joints, the pelvis contains the pubic symphysis, which unites the two pubic bones.[3]

The sacroiliac joint is a synovial joint formed by the auricular surfaces of the ilium and sacrum. The joint surfaces possess irregular elevations and depressions that interlock with similar irregularities on the opposite joint surface. This configuration limits mobility and helps to stabilize the joint.[5] With aging, the elevations and depressions increase in size and number, and fibrous adhesions between the joint surfaces develop. Thus, the joint space is gradually obliterated.[5] Additional stability is provided to the sacroiliac joints by strong ligaments, including the interosseous ligament and the anterior and posterior sacroiliac ligaments.[8] The sacrotuberous and sacrospinous ligaments connect the sacrum and ischium and help to further stabilize the joint.[8]

Movements of the Sacroiliac Joint

The sacroiliac joint is known as a very stable joint because of its bony configuration and ligamentous support. However, a small amount of movement does occur at the sacroiliac joint.[5] The direction, amount, and significance of this movement is quite controversial.

The classical movements attributed to the sacroiliac joint are nutation and counternutation.[8] Nutation is an anterior tilting of the sacrum so that the base moves anteriorly and the apex moves posteriorly. Counternutation is a return from the position of nutation. Although many sources agree on the existence of these movements, there is a great discrepancy on the location of the axis of movement and the type of movement that occurs. The motion has been described as a rotation, a translation,[8] or a combination of rotation and translation.[3] One study reports that the sacral base moves anteriorly 5 to 6 mm at the extremes of nutation.[3]

Mitchell[31] identifies three different axes of movement for sacral flexion and extension: one that occurs with respiration, one that occurs with spinal flexion and extension, and one that occurs with locomotion. He also identifies two oblique axes about which sacral torsions occur. The sacral torsions involve a rotation of the sacrum about an axis that passes diagonally through the sacrum. Other sources identify only one axis of motion in the sacroiliac joint.[3,8]

Porterfield and DeRosa[5] state that in the general population, movements of the sacroiliac joints are very small accommodating movements. They state that the focus should be on movements that develop around the sacroiliac joints rather than actual movement.

Forces Acting on the Sacroiliac Joint

The sacrum is subjected to forces that arise from the lumbar spine and above. These forces are known as trunk forces. The inominate bones are subjected to forces that pass to them through the lower extremities. These forces are known as ground forces. Trunk and ground forces converge at the sacroiliac joint and must be attenuated to prevent injury.[5] Some attenuation of forces occurs in the compression of the cartilage that lines the joint surfaces.[5]

DonTigny[32] describes a self-bracing mechanism of the sacroiliac joints that adds stability to the joints and decreases available movement. Trunk forces produce an anterior rotation of the sacrum. The anterior rotation tightens the sacrotuberous, sacrospinous, and posterior sacroiliac ligaments and locks the sacroiliac joints. On the other hand, posterior rotation of the sacrum or anterior rotation of the inominates releases the self-bracing mechanism and decreases the locking between joint surfaces.

DonTigny notes that in ambulation, one inominate can rotate anteriorly while the opposite is in posterior rotation. He states that dysfunction of the sacroiliac joints occurs when one or both inominates become stuck in anterior rotation. Although DonTigny defines this as the only type of dysfunction occurring in the sacroiliac joints, Mitchell[31] defines a number of dysfunctions, including sacral torsions, sacral flexions, iliac rotations, iliac flares, and iliac upslips.

CLINICAL APPLICATIONS

Pregnancy and Sacroiliac Sprains

During pregnancy, a hormone known as relaxin is released. This hormone increases the extensibility of the connective tissue and allows the pelvic outlet to expand during childbirth.[5] However, it also allows more movement and decreases the self-bracing mechanism of the sacroiliac joints. These changes make the sacroiliac joints more vulnerable to injury. Thus, a woman may be more susceptible to sacroiliac sprains during pregnancy and for a time after.[5]

References

1. Taylor JR, Twomey LT. Functional and applied anatomy of the cervical spine. In: Grant R, ed. *Physical Therapy of the Cervical and Thoracic Spine.* 2nd ed. New York, NY: Churchill Livingstone; 1994.
2. Panjabi MM, Krag MH, Chung TQ. Effects of disc injury on mechanical behavior of the human spine. *Spine.* 1984; 9:707.
3. Williams PL, Warwick R, eds. *Gray's Anatomy.* 36th ed. Philadelphia, Pa: WB Saunders Company; 1980.
4. Kendall FP, McCreary EK. *Muscle Testing and Function.* Baltimore, Md: Williams & Wilkins; 1983.
5. Porterfield JA, DeRosa C. *Mechanical Low Back Pain, Perspectives in Functional Anatomy.* Philadelphia, Pa: WB Saunders Company; 1991.
6. Bogduk N, Twomey LT. *Clinical Anatomy of the Lumbar Spine.* Melbourne: Churchill Livingstone; 1991.
7. Grieve GP. *Common Vertebral Joint Problems.* London: Churchill Livingstone; 1988.
8. Kapandji IA. *The Physiology of the Joints, Vol. 3, The Trunk and the Vertebral Column.* London: Churchill Livingstone; 1974.
9. Paris SV. *The Spine, Etiology and Treatment of Dysfunction including Joint Manipulation.* New Zealand: Stanley V. Paris; 1979.
10. Keim HA. Low back pain. In: Shapter RK, ed. *Clinical Symposia.* Vol 25. Summit,NJ: CIBA Pharmaceutical Company; 1973.
11. Steadman's Medical Dictionary. Baltimore, Md: Williams & Wilkins; 1976.
12. Brunnstrom S. *Clinical Kinesiology.* Philadelphia, Pa: FA Davis; 1972.
13. Porterfield JA, DeRosa C. *Mechanical Neck Pain, Perspectives in Functional Anatomy.* Philadelphia, Pa: WB Saunders Company; 1995.
14. Bogduk N. Biomechanics of the cervical spine. In: Grant R, ed. *Physical Therapy of the Cervical and Thoracic Spine.* 2nd ed. New York, NY: Churchill Livingstone Inc; 1994.
15. Adams LP, Tregidga A, Driver-Jowith JP, Selby P, Wynchank S. Analysis of motion of the head. *Spine.* 1994; 19:266-271.
16. Iai H, Goto S, Yamagata M, et al. Three-dimensional motion of the upper cervical spine in rheumatoid arthritis. *Spine.* 1994; 19:272-276.
17. Dvorak J, Antinnes JA, Panjabi M, Loustalot D, Bonomo M. Age and gender related normal motion of the cervical spine. *Spine.* 1992; 17:S393-398.
18. Alund M, Larsson SE. Three-dimensional analysis of neck motion. A clinical method. *Spine.* 1990; 15:87-91.
19. Butler DS. *Mobilisation of the Nervous System.* Melbourne: Churchill Livingstone; 1991.
20. Lee D. Biomechanics of the thorax. In: Grant R, ed. *Physical Therapy of the Cervical and Thoracic Spine.* 2nd ed. New York, NY: Churchill Livingstone; 1994.
21. Yamamoto I, Panjabi NM, Oxland TR, Crisco JJ. The role of the iliolumbar ligament in the lumbosacral junction. *Spine.* 1990; 15:1138-1141.
22. Smith TJ, Fernie GR. Functional biomechanics of the spine. *Spine.* 1991; 16:1197-1203.
23. Ahmed AM, Duncan NA, Burke DL. The effect of facet geometry on the axial torque-rotation response of lumbar motion segments. *Spine.* 1990; 15:391-401.
24. Haher TR, O'Brien M, Felmly WT, et al. Instantaneous axis of rotation as a function of the three columns of the spine. *Spine.* 1992; 17:S149-154.
25. McFadden KD, Taylor JR. Axial rotation in the lumbar spine and gapping of the zygapophyseal joints. *Spine.* 1990; 15:295-259.
26. Shirazi-Adl A. Biomechanics of the lumbar spine in sagittal lateral moments. *Spine.* 1994; 19:2407- 2414.
27. Lin RM, Yu CY, Chang ZJ, Chang CL, Su FC. Flexion-extension rhythm in the lumbosacral spine. *Spine.* 1994; 19:2204-2209.
28. Crisco JJ, Panjabi MM. The intersegmental and multisegmental muscles of the lumbar spine. A biomechanical model comparing lateral stabilizing potential. *Spine.* 1991; 16:793-799.
29. Macintosh JE, Bogduk N. The attachments of the lumbar erector spinae. *Spine.* 1991; 16:783-792.
30. Adams MA, Green TP, Dolan P. The strength in anterior bending of lumbar intervertebral discs. *Spine.* 1994; 19:2197-2203.
31. Mitchell FL, Moran PS, Pruzzo NA. *An Evaluation and Treatment Manual of Osteopathic Muscle Energy Techniques.* Valley Park, Mo: Mitchell, Moran, and Pruzzo, Associates; 1979
32. DonTigny RL. Mechanics and treatment of the sacroiliac joint. *Journal of Manual and Manipulative Therapy.* 1993; 1(3):12.

Suggested Reading

Bogduk N. Biomechanics of the cervical spine. In: Grant R, ed. *Physical Therapy of the Cervical and Thoracic Spine.* 2nd ed. New York, NY: Churchill Livingstone; 1994.

Bogduk N, Twomey LT. *Clinical Anatomy of the Lumbar Spine.* Melbourne: Churchill Livingstone; 1991.

Grieve GP. *Common Vertebral Joint Problems.* London: Churchill Livingstone; 1988.

Kapandji IA. *The Physiology of the Joints, Vol 3: The Trunk and the Vertebral Column.* London: Churchill Livingstone; 1974.

Lee D. Biomechanics of the thorax. In: Grant R, ed. *Physical Therapy of the Cervical and Thoracic Spine.* 2nd ed. New York: Churchill Livingstone; 1994.

Porterfield JA, DeRosa C. *Mechanical Low Back Pain, Perspectives in Functional Anatomy.* Philadelphia, Pa: WB Saunders Company; 1991.

Porterfield JA, DeRosa C. *Mechanical Neck Pain, Perspectives in Functional Anatomy.* Philadelphia, Pa: WB Saunders Company; 1995.

Taylor JR, Twomey LT. Functional and applied anatomy of the cervical spine. In: Grant R, ed. *Physical Therapy of the Cervical and Thoracic Spine.* 2nd ed. New York, NY: Churchill Livingstone; 1994.

1. Why should an individual with a bulging or herniated lumbar disc avoid carrying heavy loads and working in a forward bent position?

2. A doctor recommended that his patient with a bulging disc lie down for an hour several times during the course of the day. Why is this good advice?

3. Why should an individual with spondylolysis avoid carrying heavy loads?

4. An individual sprained one of the facet joints in his low back in a recent motor vehicle accident. Why should he avoid vigorous trunk rotation?

5. How does muscle strength aid in stabilizing the lumbar spine?

6. Should abdominal muscle strengthening be included in an exercise program designed to prevent low back injuries? What about iliopsoas strengthening?

7. A pregnant woman complains of low back pain whenever she tries to perform her step aerobics. What could be a possible explanation of the cause of her pain.

8. Why is there less flexion range of motion in the thoracic spine than in the cervical or lumbar spine?

9. An individual with severe forward head posture noted that he had trouble reaching overhead. How could this be related to the posture of his neck?

10. An individual injured her neck in a motor vehicle accident. Several weeks later she was diagnosed as having carpal tunnel syndrome. Could the two be related?

11. Demonstrate the adjustments that the upper cervical spine must make to place the head in a laterally flexed position.

12. What muscles help to adjust or "fine tune" the position of the head.

13. Why is the sternocleidomastoid muscle frequently injured in motor vehicle accidents?

14. Locate the curves of the cervical spine, thoracic spine, lumbar spine, and sacrum.

15. Demonstrate the gross movements of flexion, extension, lateral flexion, and rotation.

16. Compare and contrast the orientation of the facet joints in the different regions of the spine. How does this orientation affect motion?

17. Palpate the spinous processes of C2 and C7.

CHAPTER 10

THE HIP COMPLEX

Gina L. Konin, PT, ATC

OBJECTIVES

After completion of this chapter, the reader will be able to:

DIDACTIC

1. Describe the hip joint anatomy.
2. List the motions that occur at the hip joint.
3. Compare open versus closed chain movement and muscle action at the hip.
4. Describe both passive and active insufficiency that may occur at the hip.
5. Describe a Trendelenburg sign.

PRACTICAL

1. Demonstrate passive and active insufficiency at the hip.
2. Demonstrate gluteus medius weakness/Trendelenburg gait.
3. Demonstrate open and closed kinetic chain hip flexion.
4. Discuss concurrent forces at the hip joint and how they relate to gait.
5. Discuss the effects of coxa vara and coxa valga in relation to forces at the hip.

BASIC ANATOMY REVIEW

The hip is a very complex joint designed to allow for a greater extent of mobility compared to the role it plays in stability. The hip joint, similar to that of the shoulder, contains a ball and socket design and therefore has similar features. Compared to the shoulder, the hip has stronger ligamentous structures, which provide additional stability.

Various ligaments are involved in hip stability. The iliofemoral ligament, also known as the "Y" ligament, is an anteriorly strong band[1] (Figure 10-1). The Y ligament attaches to the anterior inferior iliac spine and the acetabular rim and extends to the intertrochanteric line of the femur.[1] This ligament helps to prevent hyperextension of the femur at the hip. Thus, one could stand erect without anterior hip muscle contractions.

The pubofemoral ligament arises from the inferior acetabular rim and the iliopubic eminence and blends with the medial part of the iliofemoral ligament.[1] Based on the location, the pubofemoral ligament strengthens the anterior and inferior portions of the hip joint capsule (see Figure 10-1). In addition, the pubofemoral ligament tightens during hip extension and abduction.[1]

The ischiofemoral ligament arises from the ischial portion of the acetabular rim and spirals superolaterally to the neck of the femur, medial to the base of the greater trochanter.[1] This ligament strengthens the posterior hip joint capsule. In addition, the biomechanical design tends to "screw" the femoral head medially into the acetabulum during extension of the femur. This resists hyperextension of the femur in the acetabulum.[1]

The functional anatomy of the hip includes multiple bursae. The purpose of the bursae are to decrease friction at various locations. Two bursae that are frequently injured or inflamed are the trochanteric bursa and the iliopsoas bursa. The trochanteric bursa covers the greater trochanter of the femur and is superseded by the tensor fascia lata.[2] The iliopsoas bursa is located between the articular capsule and the iliopsoas muscle on the anterior aspect of the joint.[3]

The Hip Joint

The femur and acetabulum articulate to form the actual hip joint. The joint itself is considered to be synovial and diarthrodial. This design allows for 3° of freedom of movement (flexion/extension,

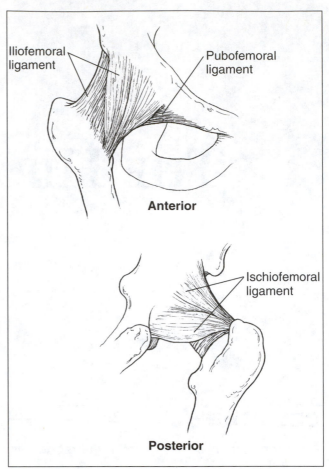

Figure 10-1. Ligaments of the hip.

abduction/adduction, and internal rotation/external rotation) (Figure 10-2). The pelvic area supports the spine and trunk in addition to transferring the weight to the lower extremities.[3] The pelvis is formed by the two innominate bones, the sacrum, and the coccyx. The two innominate bones are created by a fusion of the ilium, ischium, and pubis (see Figure 10-2).

The acetabulum is a concave hemispherical socket located on the lateral pelvis. It contains a rim and several anatomical portions. The rim of the acetabulum is lined with fibrocartilage called the acetabular labrum. This creates a deeper socket for stability of the femoral head within. The central portion of the acetabulum, termed the acetabular fossa, is nonarticular and contains a fat pad that is covered with synovial fluid.[4] The inferior portion of the acetabulum is interrupted by a deep notch called the acetabular notch.[4] The purpose of the acetabular notch is to provide a passage for the ligamentum teres to provide blood flow to the femoral head.

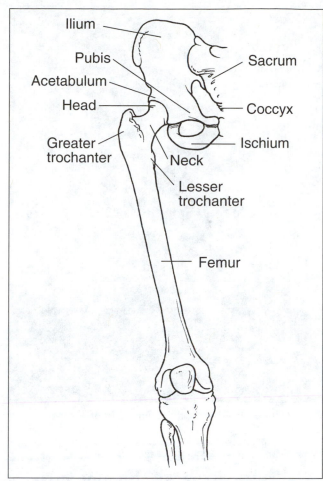

Figure 10-2. Bones of the hip joint.

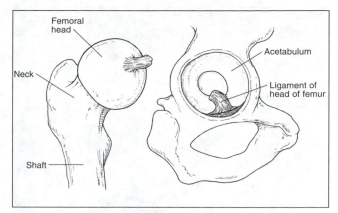

Figure 10-3. The femoral head, neck, and shaft.

more pronounced and the overall shape is more vertical and conical in the male pelvis.[5]

KINEMATIC MOTION

Motions

The hip has 3° of freedom. Flexion and extension occur in the sagittal plane through a frontal axis. Abduction and adduction occur in the frontal plane through an anterior/posterior axis. Lateral and medial, or external and internal rotation respectively, occur in a transverse plane through a vertical or longitudinal axis[6] (Figures 10-4a through 10-4c). See Table 10-1 for the normal physiological ranges of motion occurring at the hip joint.

As the hip is similar to the shoulder with respect to anatomical design, so are many of its component motions. The femoral head must glide posteriorly and inferiorly during flexion of the hip (Figure 10-5). It must glide inferiorly during abduction of the hip. External rotation of the femur in the acetabulum combines with an anterior glide of the femoral head, while internal rotation combines with a posterior glide of the femoral head.[7] These accessory motions are necessary to allow for normal physiological range of motion.

The hip is most stable in combined extension, abduction, and external rotation (closed packed position).[7] This position maximizes congruency of the joint surfaces, such as in standing. The resting position of the hip is seen with 30° of flexion, 30° of abduction, and slight external rotation.[8] The resting position provides the capsule with its greatest capacity and the joint is simultaneously under the least amount of stress.

As mentioned, the acetabular labrum deepens the surface for the femoral head to rest within. The femoral head is covered by articular cartilage for protection in the socket and attaches to the femoral neck, which connects the femoral shaft[4] (Figure 10-3). Therefore, the femur creates a lever arm for muscles and allows movement at the hip joint.

The hip joint is enclosed by a strong, dense fibrous capsule. The articular capsule forms a cylindrical sleeve that encloses the hip joint and most of the neck of the femur.[1] The capsule helps reinforce the hip joint to provide stability and helps to maintain the femoral head in the acetabulum. The synovial capsule lines the acetabular fossa and covers the fatty pad in the acetabular notch.[1] The synovial capsule also lines the internal surface of the fibrous capsule.

The male and female pelvis vary in structure and function. The female pelvis has a larger oval or round design to accommodate child birth.[5] The male pelvis is designed for speed and strength and is therefore heavier. The muscle attachments are

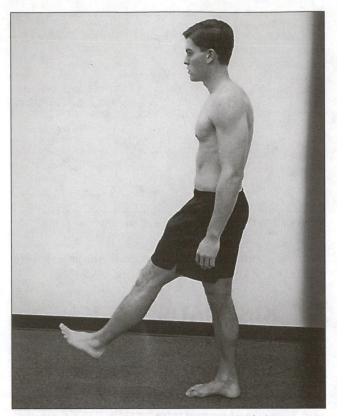

Figure 10-4a. Movements of the hip in a sagittal plane.

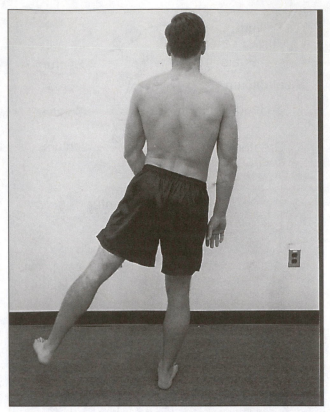

Figure 10-4b. Movements of the hip in a frontal plane.

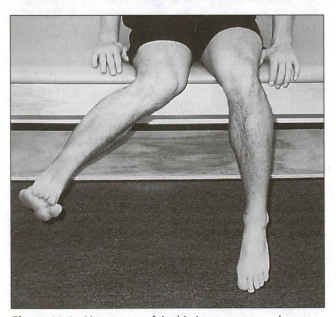

Figure 10-4c. Movements of the hip in a transverse plane.

Table 10-1
Passive Range of Hip Motion

Flexion	0 to 120°
Extension	0 to 30°
Abduction	45° to 50°
Adduction	20° to 30°
Internal roatation	0 to 35°
External rotation	0 to 45°

Open Chain versus Closed Chain

Open chain movement indicates the distal segment is moving on the stationary proximal segment. For example, in open chain hip flexion, the femur flexes on the pelvis. This would allow one to lift the foot off the floor. Closed chain movement indicates the proximal segment moves and the distal segment is stationary. Closed chain hip flexion would produce forward movement of the pelvis on a stationary femur, such as bending forward (Figures 10-6 a and 10-6b).

Open chain hip extension involves the femur moving posteriorly on a fixed pelvis. By contrast, closed chain hip extension involves the pelvis mov-

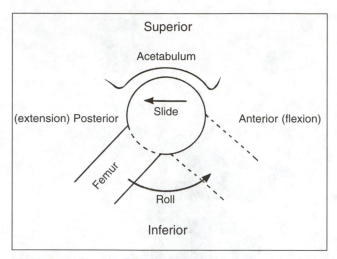

Figure 10-5. The femoral head moves posteriorly and inferiorly with hip flexion.

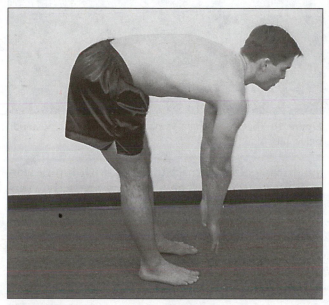

Figure 10-6b. Closed chain hip flexion.

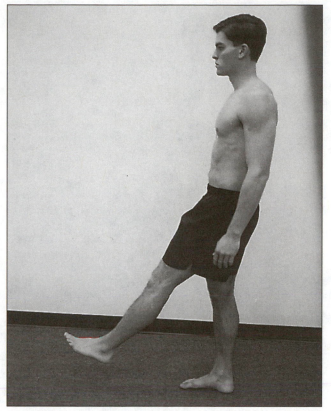

Figure 10-6a. Standing hip flexion in open chain.

terns have been extensively studied and shown to incorporate multiple open and closed chain movements in combination with concentric and eccentric muscle activity and control.

THE HIP DURING GAIT

Stance Phase

In unilateral stance, the major function of the hip abductors is to maintain a level pelvis.[6] The abductors must generate a force equal to two times the person's body weight to prevent the opposite hip from dropping.[7] If weakness of the abductors is present, the contralateral side drops (Figure 10-9). This posture during gait is termed a Trendelenburg sign. In addition, the extensors assist in controlling the hip and maintaining a level pelvis.[9] Joint compressive forces may be up to 2.5 times the body weight during single leg stance, and the weightbearing force on the femoral head is greater than body weight due to the shift of the center of gravity during single leg stance.[7,10-12]

ing posteriorly on a fixed femur. This movement would perform a posterior pelvic tilt in a standing position (Figures 10-7 a and 10-7b). Another important example of open chain versus closed chain is observed in the stance phase of gait. Open chain abduction of the hip defines the femur moving away from the midline. Closed chain abduction of the hip defines lateral flexion of the pelvis on the femur (Figure 10-8).

Many activities of daily living involve concentric and eccentric muscle actions. This includes transitions from supine to sit to stand, squatting, bending, and ambulating (Table 10-2). Gait pat-

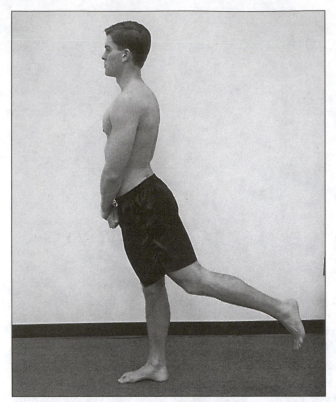

Figure 10-7a. Open chain hip extension while standing.

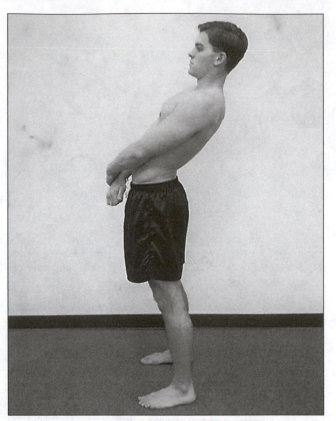

Figure 10-7b. Closed chain trunk extension with a posterior pelvic tilt.

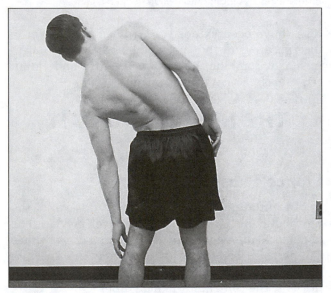

Figure 10-8. Closed chain trunk lateral flexion.

Pre-Swing Phase

Muscles of the hip are quite active during the pre-swing phase. The hip flexors contract concentrically to lift and move the leg forward. The quadriceps also contract to assist with hip flexion and knee extension. The adductors are active during the intervals of exchange between the swing phase and the stance phase and decelerate passive abduction, which occurs during the weight shift to the contralateral side.[9]

Late Mid-Swing Phase

The hamstrings contract in the late mid-swing phase eccentrically to decelerate the lower extremity. The hamstrings may limit the amount of hip flexion and knee extension if passive insufficiency is present.

Terminal Swing Phase

The adductor magnus contracts and progressively increases in intensity throughout the phase to provide hip stability.[9] The gluteus maximus action begins with the end of the terminal swing phase. Upon initial contact or heel strike, the gluteus maximus quickly contracts and increases in

Table 10-2
Muscle Activity During Movements

Action	Activity	Muscles	Method	Chain
Flexion of femur on pelvis	Lift foot march	Hip flexors	Concentric	O
Flexion of pelvis on femur	Bend at the hips or waist	Extensors*	Eccentric	C
Unilateral stance	Left leg stance	Left abductors	Concentric	C
		Left gluteus medius		
Extension of femur on pelvis	Step up	Extensors	Concentric	C
Flexion of femur on pelvis	Step down	Extensors	Eccentric	C
(The above are all performed in a standing position)				
Flexion of femur on pelvis	Knee to chest	Hip flexors	Concentric	O
Flexion of pelvis on femur	Sit up	Hip flexors	Concentric	C
		Rectus abdominal		

(The above are performed in a supine position)

*No concentric contraction is required secondary to the fact that gravity assists with flexion if beyond the center of gravity

O = open; C = closed

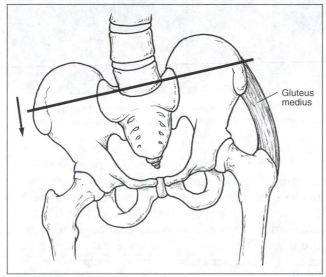

Figure 10-9. Gluteus medius weakness allows the contralateral pelvis to drop inferiorly.

intensity to counteract the loading response and to maintain a neutral posture with pelvic position.[9]

PASSIVE VERSUS ACTIVE INSUFFICIENCY

Length-tension relationships will affect strength and motion at the hip joint. Active insufficiency is demonstrated by various muscles and positions at the hip. The rectus femoris is a two-joint muscle based on its origin and insertion. The rectus femoris may experience active insufficiency when hip flexion combined with knee extension, thereby placing the muscle on slack (Figure 10-10a). This position decreases the amount of force it may generate based on the length of the muscle.

The rectus femoris may also experience passive insufficiency at the hip. Hip extension may be limited by the rectus femoris when combined with knee flexion. This position puts the rectus femoris on stretch and thus may limit hip extension. Likewise, placing the hip in a position of extension may limit the amount of available flexion at the ipsilateral knee (Figure 10-10b).

The hamstrings are also two-joint muscles. The hamstrings experience active insufficiency with combined hip extension and knee flexion.[6] This position puts the hamstrings in a shortened position to generate less force. Passive insufficiency of the hamstrings occurs during hip flexion with simultaneous knee extension. This position stretches the hamstrings, which may limit hip flexion. This is demonstrated during a straight leg raise. Therefore, to effectively stretch the hamstrings, the hip must be flexed and the knee extended. This concept can be applied to stretching of all two-joint muscles.

COMMON INJURIES TO THE HIP

Various injuries may occur at the hip based on the muscular, bony, and ligamentous configuration of the hip. One may be predisposed to injuries at

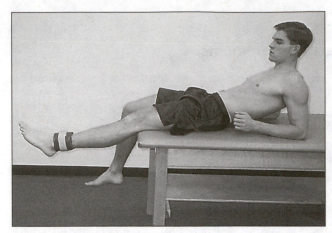

Figure 10-10a. Positions of active insufficiency with hip flexion and knee extension, both affecting the quadriceps muscle group.

the hip region due to overuse, repetition, trauma, or bony malalignment.

Bony Malalignment: Coxa Valga and Coxa Vara

Coxa valga and coxa vara correlate to the angle of inclination of the femoral head and neck with the femoral shaft. The normal angle of inclination in an adult is 125° and in a child the angle of inclination is 150°.[7] Changes in this angle affect the length-tension relationship of various hip musculature (Figure 10-11a).

Coxa valga is the increased angle of inclination between the femoral head and neck with the femoral shaft (Figure 10-11b). This increased angle decreases the efficiency of the hip abductors based on the length-tension relationship. Therefore, the abductors exert greater force to counterbalance gravity during single-leg stance of the supporting limb.[4] Increased muscle forces also increase joint compressive forces. Coxa valga reduces the magnitude of the bending movement of the head and neck on the shaft. The resultant forces act almost parallel to the axis of the head and neck.[4] Overall, coxa valga is undesirable since stability may be compromised.[13-15]

Coxa vara is a decreased angle of inclination, which creates a position of stability through an improved length-tension relationship of the abductors (Figure 10-11c). Less force is required by the abductors to counterbalance gravity during single-leg stance. Coxa vara also increases the magnitude of the bending movement of the head and neck on the femur, which may predispose femoral neck fractures or epiphyseal slippage.[15]

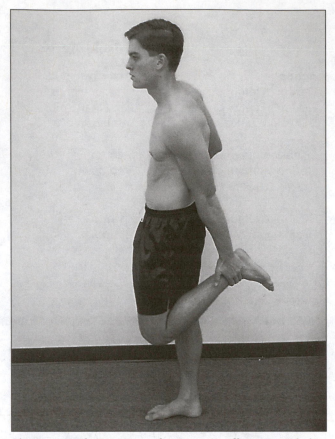

Figure 10-10b. Positions of passive insufficiency with hip extension and knee flexion, both affecting the quadriceps muscle group.

Anteversion and retroversion are variations in the angle of torsion of the femoral neck in reference to the shaft. The femoral neck is normally directed 15° anteriorly or forward[7] (Figure 10-12). In an anteverted anatomic standing position, the acetabulum and the femoral neck are focused anteriorly, causing a large portion of the articulating surface of the femoral head to not be in contact with the acetabulum. This creates a high intensity area of weightbearing force that is concentrated on a small surface area on the femoral head.[7] Ultimately, this may lead to degenerative joint disease.

Anteversion of the femoral neck has a larger angle of torsion and results in a relative medial rotation of the femur.[4] This position may predispose the hip joint to anterior dislocation.[4] Anteversion creates a "toe in" gait, and the person appears to lack external rotation.[7] Retroversion of the femoral neck has a decreased angle of torsion and results in a relative lateral rotation of the femur. This position of lateral rotation of the femur improves stability.[4] Retroversion gait appears to lack internal rotation, and the person ambulates with a "toe out" style.[7]

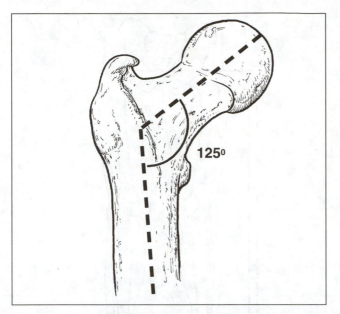

Figure 10-11a. Neck to shaft alignment of the femur: normal.

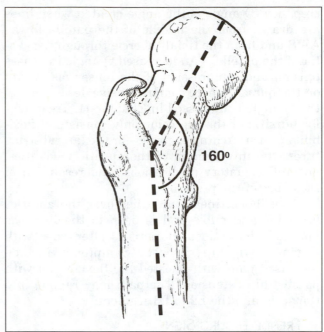

Figure 10-11b. Neck to shaft alignment of the femur: coxa valga.

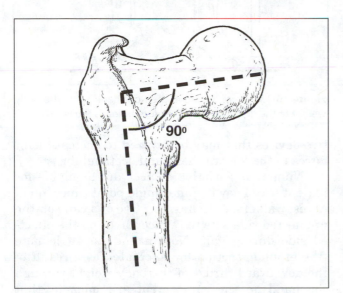

Figure 10-11c. Neck to shaft alignment of the femur: coxa.

Soft Tissue Injuries

TROCHANTERIC BURSITIS

The trochanteric bursa lies superficial and posterolateral to the greater trochanter and deep to the tensor fascia lata. This bursa may become inflamed, resulting in trochanteric bursitis.[7] This is commonly caused by tensor fascia lata tightness and/or overuse, which creates repetitive friction of the bursa.[16]

Trochanteric bursitis may also develop among those with an increased Q-angle or leg length dis-

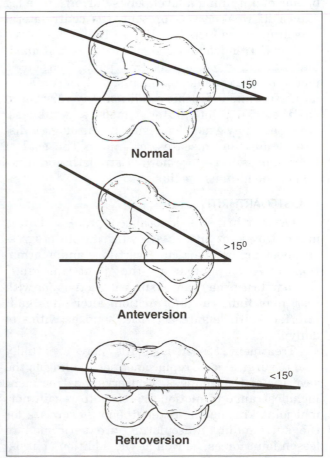

Figure 10-12. Angles of hip torsion (version): a. normal; b. anteversion; c. retroversion.

crepancy (Q-angle is the angle created when lines are drawn from the middle of the patella to the ASIS and from the tibial tubercle through the center of the patella).[3] An increased Q-angle increases tension and compression of the tensor fascia lata on the bursa. A more comprehensive description of the Q-angle is discussed in Chapter 11. Treatment for bursitis of the hip commonly consists of flexibility and stretching exercises for the lateral structures, the intervention of therapeutic modalities, anti-inflammatory medications, and resolution of the cause of the problem.

The iliopectineal bursa lies over the anterior hip joint and pubis and is deep to the iliopsoas muscle.[7] Iliopectineal bursitis is often seen with degenerative hip disease. Symptoms include increased pain with resisted hip flexion and with passive hip extension. The pain may radiate into the groin and the L2 to L3 segment.[7]

TRENDELENBURG SIGN

The Trendelenburg sign occurs with gluteus medius weakness. The gluteus medius is responsible for maintaining a level pelvis during single leg stance. If weakness is present, the contralateral side drops or adducts (see Figure 10-9). This is evident as a Trendelenburg sign during gait. If maximal adduction occurs at this point, tension is placed on the capsule, ligaments, and tensor fascia lata.[8] Treatment for this condition may vary based on the cause of gluteus medius weakness. Weakness may exist as a result of neurological diseases, muscular diseases, or injury. The goal of treatment is to restore normal strength and function of the gluteus medius.

OSTEOARTHRITIS

Osteoarthritis is a localized process that is marked by joint space narrowing due to progressive destruction of articular cartilage and a formation of osteophytes at the joint margin.[17] Osteoarthritis may cause pain with activity or with rest, may limit range of motion, alter one's gait, interfere with leisure activities, and activities of daily living.

Treatment of osteoarthritis may eventually lead to surgical joint replacement depending on the severity of the changes. Conservative treatment includes range of motion exercises to regain normal joint kinematics. Strengthening exercises for the surrounding musculature are performed to lessen joint forces, as well as the addition of assis-

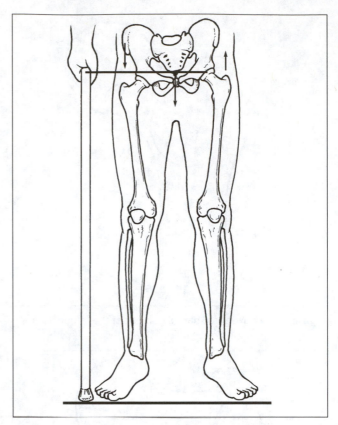

Figure 10-13. Use of a cane in the right hand shifts the body weight to the right side and therefore unloads the left hip.

tive devices that may be utilized to decrease joint forces to the femoral head and acetabulum.

Numerous assistive devices are available for patient use. They include single point canes, quad canes, walkers, crutches, etc. Use of a cane on the unaffected side acts to reduce forces on the effected side during gait. Norkin and Levangie note "the ground reaction force, created as a result of the downward thrust of the body weight through the hand on the cane, creates a moment that helps to counteract the moment created by gravity around the effected hip in unilateral stance"[4] (Figure 10-13).

Congenital Hip Dislocation

Congenital hip dislocations may be traced to faulty hip development in utero. Studies of neonates indicate that extreme hip positions in the developing fetus create more articular cartilage damage than do more moderate positions.[18] The hip does not form a fixed fulcrum of rotation about which movements may be generated, therefore the acetabulum may not fully develop, and the femoral head may not have the full spherical shape.[18]

Traumatic Hip Dislocation

Traumatic hip dislocations usually occur from a traumatic force directed along the long axis of the femur with the knee in a flexed position. The hip dislocates posteriorly and presents with hip flexion, internal rotation, and adduction.[3] This type of dislocation causes capsular and ligamentous damage. Treatment approaches to a traumatic posterior hip dislocation include strengthening of the hip extensors, external rotators, and abductors. Strengthening of theses specific muscles encourage stabilization of the femoral head in the acetabulum.

References

1. Moore KL. *Clinically Oriented Anatomy*. Baltimore, Md: Williams & Wilkins; 1985.
2. Booher JM, Thibodeau GA. *Athletic Injury Assessment*. St. Louis, Mo: Times Mirror/Mosby College Publishing; 1985.
3. Arnheim DD. *Modern Principles of Athletic Training*. St. Louis, Mo: Times Mirror/Mosby College Publishing; 1985.
4. Norkin C, Levangie P. *Joint Structure and Function: A Comprehensive Analysis*. Philadelphia, Pa: F.A. Davis Company; 1983.
5. Pratt NE. *Clinical Musculoskeletal Anatomy*. Philadelphia, Pa: JB Lippincott Co; 1991.
6. Lehmkuhl LD, Smith LK. *Brunnstrom's Clinical Kinesiology*. Philadelphia, Pa: FA Davis Company; 1983.
7. Hertling D, Kessler RM. *Management of Common Musculoskeletal Disorders. PT Principles and Methods*. 2nd ed. Philadelphia, Pa: JB Lippincott Co; 1990.
8. Kaltenborn F. *Manual Therapy for the Extremity Joints*. Oslo: Olaf Norlis Bokhandel; 1986.
9. Perry J. *Gait Analysis: Normal and Pathological Function*. Thorofare, NJ: SLACK Incorporated; 1992.
10. Inman VT. Functional aspects of the abductor muscles of the hip. *J Bone Joint Surg (Am)*. 1947; 29:2.
11. LeVeau B. *Williams and Lissner: Biomechanics of Human Motion*. 2nd ed. Philadelphia, Pa: WB Saunders; 1977.
12. Frankel VH, Nordin M. *Basic Biomechanics of the Skeletal System*. Philadelphia, Pa: Lea and Febiger; 1980.
13. Kapandji IA. *The Physiology of the Joints*. Baltimore, Md: Williams & Wilkins; 1970.
14. Singleton MD, LeVeau BF. The hip joint: stability and stress. A review. *Phys Ther*. 1975; 55:9.
15. Radin EL, Simon SR, Rose RM, et al. *Practical Biomechanics for the Orthopedic Surgeon*. New York, NY: John Wiley and Sons; 1979.
16. Sammarco G. The hip in dancers. *Medical Problems of Performing Artists*. 1987; 2:5-14.
17. Guccione A. Arthritis and the process of disablement. *Phys Ther*. 1994; 74:408-414.
18. Soderberg GL. *Kinesiology: Application to Pathological Motion*. Baltimore, Md: Williams & Wilkins; 1986.

1. Describe what happens with right unilateral stance if the right abductors are moderately weak.

2. If a person has a painful left hip, which side should you instruct him or her to use a cane? Explain why.

3. Describe anteversion and retroversion. What effect does this have on hip function?

4. Explain and demonstrate active insufficiency of the hamstrings.

5. Explain and demonstrate passive insufficiency of the rectus femoris.

6. Describe the function of the iliofemoral Y ligament.

7. Explain the muscular functions during closed chain hip flexion. Include concentric, eccentric, and stationary descriptions.

8. If a person has trochanteric bursitis secondary to tightness, what structure may be tight? Explain this relation to the trochanteric bursa.

9. Explain and demonstrate the motions at the hip joint. Be sure to include the planes and axes in which these motions occur.

10. Describe the different muscle actions occurring at the hip when performing a step-up versus a step-down.

11. If a person suffered a traumatic posterior dislocation of the hip, which muscles may need strengthening? Why?

CHAPTER 11

THE KNEE COMPLEX

Mary Mundrane-Zweiacher, PT, ATC

OBJECTIVES

After completion of this chapter, the reader will be able to:

DIDACTIC

1. Describe the two joints that make up the knee complex.
2. Identify soft tissue structures and their significance to mobility and stability.
3. Describe the structure and function of the menisci.
4. Describe the passive and active components of patellar stabilization.
5. Using the convex/concave rule, describe the motions occurring at the joint surfaces with knee flexion and extension.
6. Describe the common injuries that occur at the knee.

PRACTICAL

1. Palpate the superficial anatomy of the patellofemoral and tibiofemoral joints.
2. Measure the Q-angle and determine whether it is within normal limits.
3. Identify abnormal movement of the patella during knee flexion and extension.
4. Demonstrate closed and open kinetic chain exercises, including concentric and eccentric contractions occurring at the tibiofemoral and patellofemoral joint.

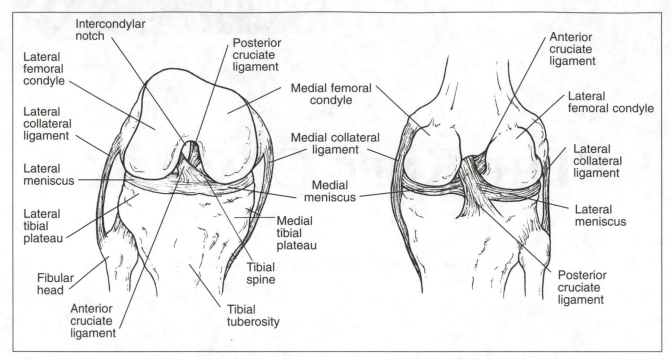

Figure 11-1. Anatomy of the knee joint.

ANATOMY

The knee joint is an integral part of the lower extremity and has to provide stability and mobility in all kinematic motions. The knee functionally consists of two separate joints: the tibiofemoral joint and the patellofemoral joint. Motion that occurs at the knee complex is a result of the interaction between the osseous and soft tissue structures of both of these joints. This interaction may be influenced by both the joints above and below and whether the motion is occurring in a closed or open kinematic chain.

Osseous Structures

THE TIBIOFEMORAL JOINT

The distal femur has two asymmetrical convex condyles that are separated by a groove called the intercondylar notch. While the femoral condyles are both convex in shape, the medial condyle s articulating surface is larger than that of the lateral condyle. The corresponding joint surfaces on the proximal tibia, or tibial plateaus, are concave with more articulating surface on the medial side as opposed to the lateral. The intercondylar notch articulates with the tibial spine. This spine is a tubercle that separates the medial and lateral tibial plateaus and serves as an attachment site for

the menisci of the knee. The spine is also important, as it appears to be a central pivot during rotation and flexion of the knee joint[1] (Figure 11-1).

Physiological angles of the knee can compare the long axis of the tibia and the long axis of the femur. This is done to identify genu varum (bow-legged) and genu valgum (knocked-knee). Both of these conditions lead to an asymmetrical loading of the femoral condyles on one side of the ipsilateral tibial plateaus. Genu valgum causes increased compression forces on the lateral compartment of the knee and increased tensile forces on the medial knee structures. Conversely, genu varum causes increased compression forces on the medial compartment of the knee and increased tensile forces on the lateral structures of the knee (Figure 11-2).

PATELLOFEMORAL JOINT

The patella is a sesamoid bone that is roughly triangular in shape and includes five distinctive ridges, referred to as facets. These facets are located and labeled as superior, inferior, lateral, medial, and odd (Figure 11-3).

There is also a central vertical ridge on the posterior aspect of the patella that follows the orientation of the trochlear groove and intercondylar groove on the anterior distal femur. The lateral aspect of a normal trochlear groove is more prominent than the medial side. A shallow sulcus, or small lateral lip, makes an individual prone to

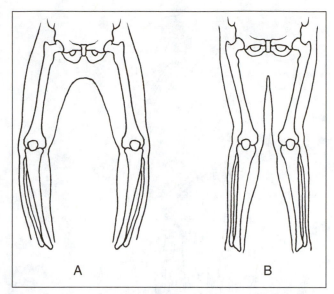

Figure 11-2. Frontal plane deviations: A. genu varum; B. genu valgum.

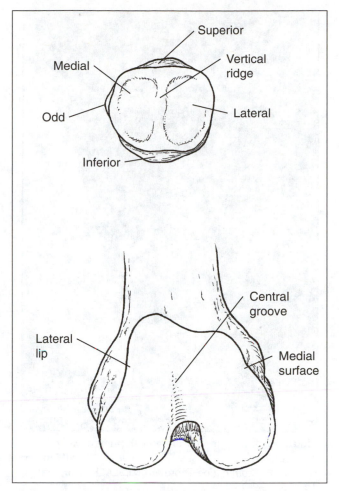

Figure 11-3. Patellofemoral joint anatomy.

patellar subluxation and dislocation, as it does not provide for a stable barrier.

The depth of the trochlear groove is determined by measuring the sulcus angle. This is an angle formed between the line from the deepest point of the femoral sulcus to the top of the medial femoral condyle, and a line from the same point on the sulcus to the top of the lateral femoral condyle. Research has shown the average sulcus angle in the normal population is 114°.[2] However, in persons who chronically dislocate in a lateral direction, the angle has been shown to increase to 127°. The posterior surface of the patella is covered with hyaline cartilage to protect the underlying subchondral bone and provide smooth movement. The patella's superior aspect, or base, is attached to the quadriceps tendon while the inferior aspect, or apex, is attached to the patellar tendon. The patellar tendon, though connecting the bony patella to the tibial tubercle of the tibia bone, is often referred to as the patellar ligament.

A measurement of the angle between the line of the quadriceps (ASIS to the midpoint of the patella) and the line of the patella tendon (midpoint of the patella to the tibial tuberosity) is called the Q-angle[2] (Figure 11-4). The average Q-angle is 12° to 13° for males and 15° to 18° for females.[3,4]

The Q-angle is generally greater in females, secondary to the wider pelvis needed for childbirth. This increased Q-angle may be associated with patellofemoral dysfunctions such as chondromalacia and subluxation or dislocation. An increased Q-angle is often seen with other malalignments such as femoral anteversion, genu valgum, a laterally situated tibial tuberosity, and external tibial torsion. By contrast, a decreased Q-angle may lead to dysfunction such as patellar tendonitis and chondromalacia.

Static Q-angles are measured in supine or nonweightbearing, and dynamic Q-angles are measured in standing. With standing, Q-angles are more relevant because the positioning is more functional. On average, the dynamic Q-angle will be greater than the static Q-angle because of the influence of foot mechanics.

Functions of the Patella

The patella has many distinct functions within the knee joint. The patella protects the anterior knee structures from trauma by covering these structures. Normal alignment allows for the quadriceps to be centralized, which in turn improves the muscles' mechanical advantage when action occurs at the knee joint. The patella also converts some compressive forces from the

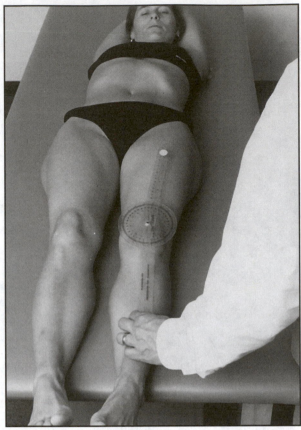

Figure 11-4. Q-angle measurement (reprinted with permission from Konin JG, Wiksten DL, Isear, Jr JA. *Special Tests for Orthopedic Examination.* Thorofare, NJ: SLACK Incorporated; 1997).

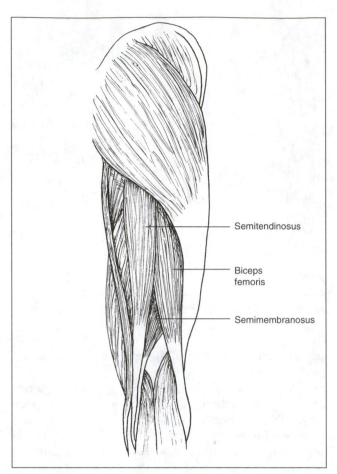

Figure 11-5. Hamstring musculature.

tibiofemoral joint into tensile forces through the patella tendon. Yet, the primary function of the patella is to improve the lever arm of the quadriceps and reduce the vector force needed to concentrically extend and eccentrically flex the knee. Persons who have had their patella removed, a process known as a patellectomy, will have a 15% to 49% reduction in the capability to extend the knee.[5-6]

Muscles

The two major muscle groups acting at the knee are the hamstrings and quadriceps. The hamstrings include the biceps femoris, semimembranosus, and semitendinosus muscles. Generally, this muscle group acts to flex the knee. However, other functions may occur. For example, since these muscles (except for the short head of the biceps femoris) attach on the ischial tuberosity, they will assist with hip extension to a significant degree. The semimembranosus and semitendi-nosus muscles will also create open chain tibial internal rotation and closed chain femoral external rotation in conjunction with the popliteus muscle as a result of their distal attachments (Figure 11-5). The average range of motion at the knee is approximately 140° of flexion, which is limited by soft tissue approximation.

The quadriceps muscle group includes the rectus femoris, vastus medialis, vastus intermedius, and vastus lateralis. Furthermore, the vastus medialis contains a separate functional part called the vastus medialis obliquus (VMO).[7-8] Together, these muscles form the extensor mechanism for the knee. The four major quadriceps muscles produce knee extension, while the rectus femoris assists with hip flexion. This is due to its origin on the anterior inferior iliac spine (Figure 11-6). Normal extension can be measured to 0° with an accompanying bone-to-bone end feel. It is possible to have range of motion in extension greater than this, which is referred to as hyperextension. Hyperextension may lead to clinical pathology, as it can interfere with normal biomechanics.

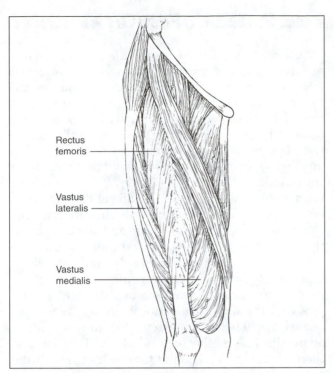

Figure 11-6. Quadriceps musculature.

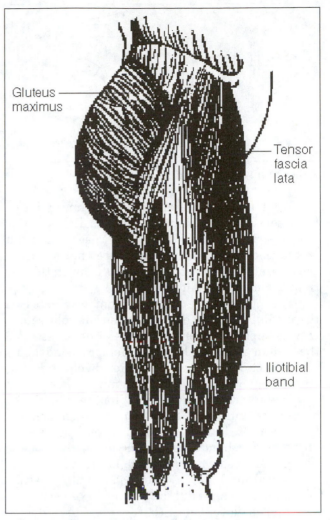

Figure 11-7. Gluteus maximus and tensor fascia latae forming the iliotibial band.

Likewise, abnormal biomechanics may lead to a hyperextension type of injury. While all four quadriceps muscles contract throughout knee extension, the specific balance of firing may vary depending on joint function. This helps to provide for optimal patella function.

Other muscles that act around the knee joint include the sartorius, gracilis, adductor magnus, gluteus maximus, tensor fascia latae, gastrocnemius, and plantaris muscles. The sartorius primarily flexes the hip but also assists with knee flexion and tibial internal rotation by pulling on its medial tibial attachment to the tibia. Likewise, the gracilis aids in knee flexion in addition to its main function as a hip adductor. The adductor magnus does not directly affect knee function since it attaches on the adductor tubercle of the femur, thus not crossing the knee joint. However, the VMO fibers originate partly from this muscle.[7] Thus, facilitation or inhibition of the adductor magnus may affect functioning of the VMO and consequently influence patellofemoral mechanics.

The gluteus maximus and tensor fascia latae come together to form a common tendon called the iliotibial band (ITB) (Figure 11-7). The ITB runs along the lateral knee and contains some fibers that interdigitate with the lateral retinaculum surrounding the knee capsule. The significance of this attachment will be discussed in more detail later in this chapter. The gastrocnemius and plantaris muscles contribute to knee flexion since they have an attachment on the posterior femur. They mildly assist the hamstring muscles, especially during closed chain activities.

Ligamentous Structures

The ligament support of the tibiofemoral joint is provided by the medial collateral ligament (MCL), the lateral collateral ligament (LCL), anterior cruciate ligament (ACL), and the posterior cruciate ligament (PCL) (see Figure 11-1 and Figure 11-8). The MCL crosses the joint on the medial aspect and resists valgus forces that are applied to the knee. The medial collateral also has some deep fibers that actually penetrate the joint capsule to blend in with the medial meniscus.

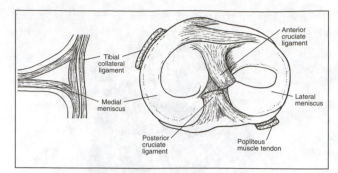

Figure 11-8. Ligamentous structures of the knee.

The lateral collateral crosses the knee joint on the lateral side and is extracapsular. Its main role is to resist varus stresses to the knee. Because it has no capsular penetration, it does not attach to the lateral meniscus. In general, it is much thinner than the medial collateral.

The anterior cruciate ligament originates on the medial, anterior aspect of the tibial plateau. It travels superior, lateral, and posterior to insert on the medial aspect of the lateral femoral condyle. Its main function is to resist anterior displacement or translation of the tibia on the femur.

The anterior cruciate is anatomically designed quite differently from the other main ligaments of the knee. It is comprised of three bands:[9] an anteromedial band that is taut when the knee is flexed and loose when the knee is extended; a posterolateral band that is loose or slack in the position of knee flexion and taut during knee extension; and an intermediate band that serves to link the anteromedial and posterolateral bands together.

The anterior cruciate also has some secondary functions about the knee. When the collateral ligaments are compromised from an injury, the ACL may help to resist excessive tibial internal rotation, as well as serve as a check for varus and valgus forces to the knee.

The posterior cruciate ligament crosses the tibiofemoral joint, originating behind the ACL attachment on the tibia. The PCL then comes superiorly and anteriorly to insert on the lateral aspect of the medial femoral condyle behind the ACL. The primary function of the posterior cruciate ligament is to resist posterior displacement or translation of the tibia on the femur. The PCL contains two portions or bands: an anterior portion that is taut during flexion of the knee, and a posterior portion that is taut during extension.[10] While the PCL limits tibial posterior displacement on the femur, especially during knee flexion, it is also a secondary restraint to varus and valgus forces.

THE PATELLOFEMORAL JOINT

Patellar stability in the trochlear groove is primarily dependent upon the connecting static and dynamic structures about the joint. As mentioned earlier, the lateral lip of the trochlear groove should be more prominent so it can serve as an osseous block to patellar subluxation and dislocation. The medial retinaculum is a thickening in the medial aspect of the fibrous capsule that runs from the patella to the medial collateral ligament. This retinaculum passively resists lateral displacement of the patella. The fibrous capsule that encloses the tibiofemoral joint is extensive and also supports the patellofemoral joint. Several muscles that are relevant to the patellofemoral dynamic stabilization interdigitate with the capsule.

The extensor mechanism of the knee is comprised of the quadriceps muscle group. When the quadriceps femoris contracts, the line of pull is along the line of the femoral shaft. This force is then imparted to the tibial tuberosity through the patella and patellar tendon. Unfortunately, the patellar tendon attachment on the tibial tuberosity is lateral to the midline of the patella, resulting in a lateral pull on the patella. This is augmented by the lateral retinaculum and the greater pull of the vastus lateralis over the other vasti musculature. The lateral retinaculum includes fibers from the ITB; thus a tight ITB may increase the lateral movement of the patella since the ITB is pulled posteriorly when the knee is flexed.

The only dynamic medial stabilizer of the knee is the vastus medialis obliquus. The VMO is active throughout full knee extension, however, its primary purpose is to counteract the pull of the lateral active and passive stabilizers of the joint.[6] Those who present with patella subluxation often exhibit a decrease in the activity of the VMO as compared to the vastus lateralis.[13-14]

ACCESSORY SOFT TISSUE STRUCTURES

The tibiofemoral joint contains two menisci that attach on the tibial plateaus, medially and laterally (see Figure 11-9). A small ligament, the coronary ligament, serves to connect these ligaments to the surface of the plateaus. The medial meniscus has a more extensive coronary ligament attachment, and as mentioned earlier, has a partial attachment to the medial collateral ligament. The

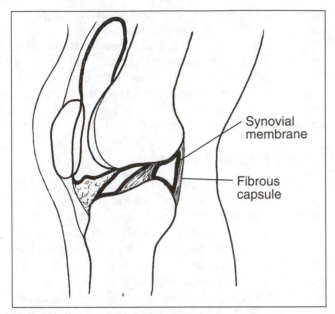

Figure 11-9. The knee joint capsule.

medial and lateral meniscus are asymmetrical in shape. The medial meniscus is semilunar in shape (C-shaped) and more narrow anteriorly than posteriorly. The medial meniscus also contains deep capsular ligaments to the femur called meniscofemoral ligaments.

The lateral meniscus, on the other hand, is more circular in shape (O-shaped). It has an attachment posterior to the popliteus muscle and may attach to the posterior cruciate ligament through the meniscofemoral ligament of Humphry and Wrisberg. The lateral meniscus has weaker coronary ligaments than the medial meniscus, insubstantial capsular ligaments, and does not attach to the lateral collateral ligament. As a result of its weaker attachments, the lateral meniscus is more mobile and less prone to injury.[15] The anterior horns, or components, of both menisci are joined by a transverse ligament.

The menisci have three primary functions at the tibiofemoral joint: stability, nutritional lubrication, and shock absorption. Joint stability occurs since the menisci form a fossa for the superiorly situated convex femoral condyles. This is enhanced since the concave menisci, although fairly thin centrally, become thicker toward the periphery. This forms a rim, or barrier, that helps to control translation about the joint. Research has shown that while the anterior cruciate ligament is the primary restraint to anterior tibial translation, the menisci may serve as secondary stabilizers.[16-17] Furthermore, cadaveric knees have been found to

have increased rotary instability following meniscal resection.[10,17]

The menisci serve to lubricate the tibiofemoral joint and thus reduce the coefficient of friction between the two articulating surfaces. The coefficient of friction (the ratio between the force necessary to move one surface horizontally over another surface and the pressure between the two surfaces) is relatively low in the knee.[18] However, MacConnaill has shown that a meniscectomy has resulted in a 20% increase in the knee joint's coefficient of friction.[19] The menisci also direct the flow of synovial fluid within the joint capsule so that optimal amounts exist between the tibial and femoral surfaces.[19] This movement of synovial fluid also helps to distribute the nutritious substances needed to supply intracapsular structures of synovial joints.

Shock absorption occurs because the menisci distribute the tensile, compressive, and rotary forces involved with weightbearing. This helps to prevent excessive loading on the articular cartilage surrounding the femur and tibia. When menisci are removed, as in meniscectomy surgery, the contact area of the joint decreases while the same forces remain present. This will subsequently increase the amount of force per unit area leading to earlier degradation of the hyaline cartilage and joint surfaces.[20-21]

The neurovascular supply to the menisci is limited. The menisci themselves have no peripheral nerve endings, making injury to these structures pain-free, except for the surrounding structures that may be involved. The blood supply to the peripheral 10% to 20% of the menisci is through the genicular arteries. The central surfaces of the menisci receive their nutrition through the synovial fluid. The peripheral portions maintain a better healing potential following injury as a result of greater nutritional capacity.

The fibrous capsule generally encloses the tibiofemoral joint structures (Figure 11-9) except the patella and cruciate ligaments. The capsule attaches on the tibia anterior to the anterior cruciate ligaments, thus the cruciate ligaments are extra-capsular. During development of the synovial capsule, pouches form and fuse in a thickening manner. These fused lines are referred to as plicae. Three plicae commonly present about the knee: suprapatellar, medial, and infrapatellar. While considered to be normal anatomy, some individuals may have excessively thickened plicae that may lead to pathology, especially when combined with poor patellofemoral mechanics.

Bursae about the knee are pouches that contain synovial fluid and serve to decrease the friction of structures about the joint. Two of the most prominent bursae are the suprapatellar bursa (located between the femur and quadriceps tendon) and the prepatellar bursa (located on the anterior aspect of the patella). The bursae are most commonly injured by a direct blow or excessive pressure, such as with repetitive kneeling. A posterior bursa also exists between the semimembranous tendon and the gastrocnemius medial tendon. Often, this bursa will become inflamed, and the observable and palpable effusion is called a baker's cyst.

An infrapatellar fat pad has been anatomically identified between the patellar tendon and the tibia. The fat pad has a good neurovascular supply. As a result, injury to this area can be quite painful. This structure is often irritated with poor patellar mechanics or by means of a contusion. This structure may also become hypertrophied or fibrotic following prolonged immobilization.

OSTEOKINEMATIC MOTION

Tibiofemoral Joint

Tibiofemoral motion can occur in all three planes, although active range of motion exists only in the sagittal and horizontal planes. Flexion and extension are actions in the sagittal plane about a frontal axis. The normal range is considered to be from full extension to about 140° of flexion.[18] Flexion is normally limited by soft tissue approximation of the gastrocsoleus musculature on the posterior thigh musculature. Extension is limited by the bony configuration of the tibiofemoral joint.

This joint is defined as a modified hinge joint since some slight rotation also occurs here. Rotation is actually a requirement for normal terminal extension to occur. When the knee is fully extended (its closed pack position), no rotation can occur. Maximum congruency exists between the intercondylar notch and the tibial spine. In addition, the menisci are compressed between the bony surfaces. As motion progresses from full extension to flexion, tibial rotation is allowed to occur.[18] Approximately 45° of external rotation and 30° of internal rotation is the maximum range allowed. This range will decrease once the knee flexes beyond 90°, since soft tissue structures will become taut.[18] Tibial rotation needs to occur in certain physical and sporting activities to allow for pivoting and cutting type movements.

Abduction and adduction are only passive motions at the tibiofemoral joint. The range of these motions are small but are best exhibited during varus and valgus controlled stressing. Functionally, abduction and adduction may occur when the tibia is in unilateral standing.

Patellofemoral Joint

The patella must also follow certain movement patterns with tibiofemoral flexion and extension. From full extension to approximately 20° of flexion, the patella moves medially off the lateral aspect of the trochlear groove. The patella then sits down in the groove in its most stable position. As knee flexion increases, the patella continues to move with varying degrees of articular surface contact. From 90° to 135° of flexion, the patella rotates along the longitudinal axis until the medial femoral condyle is in contact with the ridge that separates the medial and odd facets. Near full flexion, the patella shifts laterally to engage the odd facet against the medial femoral condyle.[22-23]

ARTHROKINEMATICS

The tibiofemoral arthrokinematics involve rolling, spinning, and gliding. Motion here will depend on whether the tibia is fixed (closed chain) or free (open chain). The femoral condylar surface is much longer than the tibial plateau surface, thus roll and glide must occur together to prevent the femur from rolling off of the tibia (Figure 11-10).

When performing a knee extension from a seated position, the concave surface of the tibial plateau moves on the convex femoral condyles. Roll and glide move in the same direction of the segment. This also occurs when the knee begins to extend. Here, the tibia must rotate externally to make up for the differences between the medial and lateral joint surfaces. Remember, the medial femoral condylar surface is longer than the lateral; therefore, external rotation must occur about the lateral meniscus to maintain articular contact while the medial condyle is still rolling. This rotation at the end range of knee extension, which locks the knee into a closed pack position, is referred to as the *screw home mechanism*. The knee unlocks and unscrews itself in the open chain as the popliteus contracts, thus internally rotating the tibia on the femur.[15]

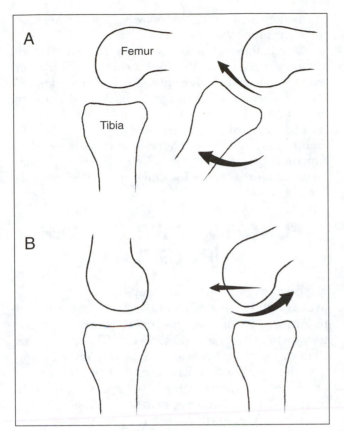

Figure 11-10. Arthrokinematics of the tibiofemoral joint: A. open chain; B. closed chain.

When the tibia is fixed and the knee is fully extended in the standing position, the femur externally rotates to unlock the knee.[15] In this situation, the convex femoral condyles move on the concave tibial surfaces, whereby rolling and gliding will occur in opposite directions of the segment. As flexion continues, the femoral condyles then begin to roll posteriorly on the tibial plateau surface, and a glide occurs in the anterior direction. The reverse occurs when the knee goes from flexion to extension in the closed chain.

During tibiofemoral range of motion, the menisci cannot remain stationary. The shape of the menisci maintain the joint congruity by providing a fossa for the femoral condyles. The menisci have to move to ensure optimal contact with the femoral articulating surface. With knee extension, the menisci move anteriorly. Here, the meniscofemoral ligaments are pulled forward by the quadriceps muscles.[15] During knee flexion, the menisci move posteriorly. The menisci also move in response to the femoral rotation that occurs with the screw home mechanism. Abnormal amounts of movement of the menisci may lead to impingement type symptoms in the knee and ultimately result in meniscal tears.

Patellofemoral Joint

The patella needs to glide in the trochlear groove to allow for normal tibiofemoral flexion and extension to occur. In addition, patella gliding assists with the moment arm of the quadriceps. When the knee flexes, the tibia moves posteriorly, placing the patella tendon in a taut position. When this happens, the patella glides distally in the trochlear groove.[14] With tibiofemoral extension, the quadriceps contraction pulls the patella proximally along the trochlear groove.[14] The patella may also glide laterally, as in the case of imbalances between active and passive stabilizing components of the patellofemoral joint.

Relationship to Other Joints

The arthrokinematics of the knee are affected by the motions of the hip, ankle, and foot. Compensations for various hip, ankle, and foot pathologies may be accomplished by altering normal knee mechanics. For example, prolonged pronation of the subtalar and midtarsal joints of the foot may lead to excessive internal rotation of the tibia.[23] The femur may then follow the tibia and internally rotate, leading to an increase in the Q-angle and a lateral drift of the patella. When this occurs, the benefits of normal torque conversion and shock absorption that occur in normal gait are lost.[23-24]

ACTIVE AND PASSIVE INSUFFICIENCY

Several two-joint muscles cross the tibiofemoral joint. Therefore, the position of the hip is a determining factor with respect to the function of the knee. When the hip is fully flexed, the proximal attachment of the rectus femoris is on slack, allowing for elongation to occur across the knee joint when moving into a flexed direction. Moving the hip into a more neutral or extended position will then elongate the rectus femoris about the hip joint, resulting in a decrease in available knee flexion. Passive insufficiency is thus illustrated when knee flexion is limited as a result of hip extension.[18]

Strength of the quadriceps, hamstrings, and the gastrocnemius may all be influenced when both joints that the muscles cross have placed the respective muscle in a shortened position. When this occurs, no longer will the muscle be able to work at its optimal length-tension relationship, thus reducing the amount of torque production.[18]

FORCES

As the patellar movement pattern varies from extension to flexion, the contact areas on the retropatellar surface also vary. During full extension, no contact exists at the patellofemoral joint. Contact begins on the inferior portion of the patella at a point between 10° and 20° of knee flexion.[1] As the flexion angle increases, contact moves superiorly, with the total contact area being approximately 2.0 cm, 3.1 cm, and 4.7 cm at 30°, 60°, and 90° of knee flexion, respectively.[1] No contact occurs at the odd facet on the medial side of the patella until approximately 135° of knee flexion.

Patellofemoral joint reaction forces (PFJRF) are those forces that occur between the two articulating surfaces of the joint. The sum of the PFJRF is equal and opposite to the resultant forces of the patella tendon and the quadriceps.[22] As the angle used to calculate the resultant force decreases with increasing knee flexion, the PFJRF increases. Therefore, the quadriceps need to exert more torque to overcome the flexion movement of the body. Reilly and Martens have shown PFJRF to be 0.5 x the amount of normal body weight forces during normal walking, 3.3 x body weight during stair climbing, and 7.8 x normal body weight forces during a squatting activity.[25]

The PFJRF can be reduced on the retropatellar surface by increasing the contact surface area. This simply allows for forces to be dissipated over a larger area.[26] As the knee joint angle changes, an inverse relationship exists between the PFJRF and the contact forces.[26] For example, as knee flexion increases, the PFJRF increases and contact forces decrease. This has clinical significance during rehabilitation exercises. Clinicians may develop different programs of quadriceps strengthening for a patellofemoral dysfunctional patient based on one of two primary rationales: first, some clinicians might strengthen the quadriceps femoris muscle in a range from 60° to 90° of knee flexion since the joint reaction forces are distributed over a larger contact surface area. Other clinicians may opt to strengthen the quadriceps muscle group when the knee is closer to terminal extension, since this has

been identified as an angle where joint reaction forces are reduced.

Patellofemoral joint reaction forces are not always consistent in all weightbearing activity. For example, Flynn and Soutas-Little have demonstrated decreased PFJRF with backward running as opposed to forward running.[27] With this in mind, backward controlled running may be beneficial in treating those who have patellofemoral dysfunctions by strengthening the quadriceps musculature under settings in which a reduced force is the outcome.

FUNCTION OF THE KNEE DURING GAIT

During gait, the quadriceps muscles are the primary stabilizers of the knee joint. From initial to terminal swing, the quadriceps contract concentrically to actively extend the knee. The quadriceps then contract eccentrically to control knee flexion from heel strike to initial swing. The hamstrings begin to contribute when the speed of gait is increased, as in running, or when an individual is going uphill. Squatting requires eccentric contractions from the quadriceps, gluteus maximus, and proximal hamstrings; while returning to the standing position from a squat requires concentric contractions from each of these same muscles. In erect standing, minimal contraction of the rectus femoris is actually required because the knee flexion/extension axis is posterior to the line of gravity.

COMMON INJURIES TO THE KNEE

Ligamentous Injuries

The knee is vulnerable to injury, as the joint surfaces are relatively shallow and serve to separate the body's largest segments. Consequently, the knee is prone to injuries from outside forces and muscle imbalances. Traumatic injuries can result from straight plane or rotary forces.

Sprains to the knee are rather common occurrences. An isolated medial collateral ligament sprain can occur when an individual's foot is fixed while a simultaneous valgus force is applied to the knee. For example, this occurs when a football

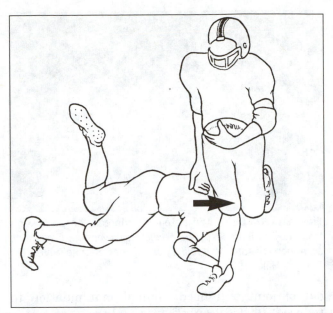

Figure 11-11. Mechanism of injury for medial collateral ligament tear.

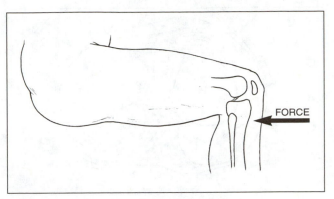

Figure 11-12. Mechanism of injury for a posterior cruciate ligament tear.

player's leg is planted and an opponent falls on the outside of his knee (Figure 11-11). The same type of injury may also occur in a motor vehicle accident (MVA) when a seat-belted driver is broadsided and his door is driven into his left knee while his foot is caught on the brake or accelerator. The MCL can also be injured indirectly when a valgus force is applied while the tibia is externally rotated. An example of this is a skier whose ski gets caught in the snow while his tibia abducts and externally rotates.

An isolated lateral collateral ligament sprain primarily occurs through a direct contact varus force that is applied to the knee while the foot is fixed. A soccer player may have this injury if an opponent's slide tackle contacts his medial knee instead of the ball. This injury is typically much less common, since the geography of the knee is less conducive to outside varus forces.

A common injury seen is a sprained anterior cruciate ligament. The anatomical structure of the ACL predisposes it to become susceptible to injury through both contact and noncontact mechanisms. A contact injury may occur when an outside force places the knee in a position of hyperextension. Here, the ACL is pulled taut and sheared. A non-contact injury is often seen when a running athlete stops quickly (rapid deceleration) or cuts laterally while his foot is planted. This creates a valgus positioning of the knee while the tibia is externally rotated about the femur.[15,28] An audible pop is often experienced by the person.

A sprain to the posterior cruciate ligament is not as common as that of the ACL. The mechanism of injury is most often a posterior force to the proximal tibia with the knee in 70° to 90° of flexion. This is seen quite frequently in MVAs in which a passenger is driven into the dashboard upon impact (Figure 11-12).

Treatments for ligament injuries to the knee vary widely. Some require operative intervention, while others may enable a person to function effectively with minimal or no discomfort at all.

Since these ligaments function to provide stability to the knee joint, rehabilitation following injuries to any of these structures should not only include strengthening to help restore normal mechanics, but also proprioceptive training.

Meniscal Injuries

Menisci may become torn either through a traumatic event or from repetitive stresses. When traumatically induced, the mechanism is usually compression and rotation of the tibiofemoral joint while the foot is fixated to a surface. This can present with a variety of types of tears, from small to large (Figure 11-13). Meniscal tears that occur over time are due to repetitive stresses. It is not accurate to label these nontraumatic, as microtrauma truly does occur. The process simply takes longer. The significance of these types of degenerative tears is that a person is likely to also have paralleled surrounding tissue damage. In fact, undetected or late detected degenerative tears may eventually predispose one to early articular cartilage damage.

Only 4% of meniscal tears can be treated successfully through conservative means, therefore surgical intervention is often indicated.[29] Treatment for the meniscal tears, operative or non-operative, will also vary widely from clinician to

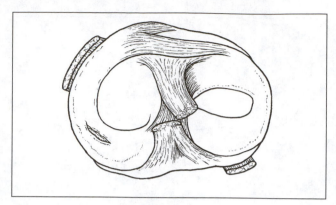

Figure 11-13. Example of a meniscal tear.

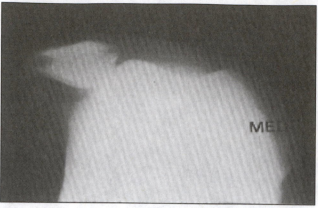

Figure 11-14. Dislocated patella (reprinted with permission from Roy S, Irvin R. *Sports Medicine: Prevention, Evaluation, Management, and Rehabilitation.* Upper Saddle River, NJ: Prentice Hall; 1983).

clinician. Regardless, sound principles that incorporate biomechanical forces and joint motions should be utilized to restore premorbid function.

Chondramalacia is defined as a softening or fissuring of the hyaline cartilage; when it occurs on the posterior surface of the patella it is chondramalacia. Hyaline cartilage receives nutrition through compression; therefore, when compression is either extremely excessive or deficient, the cartilage is subject to degradation. Hyaline cartilage is also aneural, resulting in one s inability to perceive discomfort until complete breakdown and eventual subchondral bone involvement.

Osteoarthritis is a nonsystemic disease process that leads to cartilage degeneration. The cause of osteoarthritis may be trauma, illness, or idiopathic in nature. Studies have shown that obesity may increase the chances of acquiring this condition, as joint forces are increased.[15] Osteoarthritic joints may become quite painful and swollen and eventually lead to a deterioration of function. Treatment involves strengthening of surrounding musculature and restoring joint mechanics. However, on many occasions, joint deterioration may be so exhausted that a joint arthroplasty may be indicated. Implantation of a prosthetic device allows for the creation of new joint surfaces. However, one must continue to rehabilitate to regain joint strength, flexibility, and function following surgical intervention.

Patella Subluxation and Dislocation

A patella dislocation can result from a direct blow to the patella or more typically, when one is decelerating and switching direction. The majority of the time, the patella is misplaced laterally from the trochlear groove. The patella itself may spontaneously reduce (subluxation), or it will remain out of joint and need manual manipulation to reduce it (dislocation) (Figure 11-14).

While this is typically considered to be a traumatic incident, many times predisposing factors exist that make one more prone to acquiring this problem. Muscle imbalances, large Q-angles, osseous deformities, and soft tissue restrictions are just a few of the underlying conditions that can lead to a patella displacement. Consequently, as a means of prevention as well as treatment, the structure that leads to the problems should be addressed to help restore normal alignment and function of the patellofemoral joint.

References

1. Goodfellow J, Hungerford DS, Zindel M. Patellofemoral joint mechanics and pathology. I. Functional anatomy of the patellofemoral joint. *J Bone Joint Surg.* 1976; 58B:287.
2. Larson RL. The Patella compression syndrome: surgical treatment by lateral retinacular release. *Clin Orthop.* 1978; 34:158.
3. Magee D. *Orthopedic Physical Assessment.* Philadelphia, Pa: WB Saunders Company; 1987.
4. Woodland LH, Francis RS. Parameters and comparison of the quadriceps angle of college-aged men and women in the supine and standing positions. *Am J Sports Med.* 1992; 20(2):208-211.
5. Peoples RE, Margo MK. Function after patellectomy. *Clin Orthop.* 1978; 132:180-186.
6. Sutton FS, Thompson CH, Lupke J, Kettelkamp DB. The effect of patellectomy on knee function. *J Bone Joint Surg.* 1976; 58:537-540.
7. Bose K, Kangasuntherum R, Osman M. Vastus medialis oblique: An anatomical and physiologic study. *Orthopedics.* 1980; 3:880-883.
8. Lieb FJ, Perry J. Quadriceps Function: an anatomical and mechanical study using amputated limbs. *J Bone Joint Surg.* 1968; 50A(8):1535-1548.
9. Girgis FG, Marshall JL, Monajem ARS. The cruciate ligament of the knee joint. *Clin Orthop.* 1975; 106:216.

10. Wang CJ, Walker PS, Wolf B. Rotary laxity of the human knee joint. *J Bone Joint Surg.* 1974; 56A:161.

11. Muller W. *The Knee: Form, Function and Ligament Reconstruction.* Berlin: Springer-Verlag; 1982.

12. Hutter CG, Scott W. Tibial torsion. *J Bone Joint Surg.* 1949; 31A:511.

13. Mariani D, Caruso I. An electromyelographic investigation of subluxation of the patella. *J Bone Joint Surg.* 1979; 61:169-171.

14. Hungerford DS, Barry M. Biomechanics of the patellofemoral joint. *Clin Orthop.* 1979; 9(15):144.

15. Greenfield BH. *Rehabilitation of the Knee: A Problem Solving Approach.* Philadelphia, Pa: FA Davis; 1993.

16. Levy IM, Torzilli PA, Warren RF. The effect of medial meniscectomy on the anterior-posterior motion of the knee. *J Bone Joint Surg.* 1982; 64A:883.

17. Tapper EM, Hoover HW. Late results after meniscectomy. *J Bone Joint Surg.* 1969; 51A:517.

18. Norkin CC, Levangie PK. *Joint Structure and Function: A Comprehensive Analysis.* 2nd ed. Philadelphia, Pa: FA Davis; 1991.

19. MacConnaill MA. The function of intra-articular cartilage with special reference to the knee and inferior radioulnar joints. *J Anat.* 1932; 66:210.

20. Fairbanks TJ. Knee joint changes after meniscectomy. *J Bone Joint Surg.* 1948; 30B:664.

21. Radin EL, de Lamotte F, Maquet P. Role of the menisci in the distribution of stress in the knee. *Clin Orthop.* 1984; 185:290.

22. Ficat RP, Hungerford DS. *The Patellofemoral Joint.* Baltimore, Md: Williams & Wilkins; 1977.

23. Donatelli R. *The Biomechanics of the Foot and Ankle.* Philadelphia, Pa: FA Davis; 1990.

24. Powers C, Maffucci R, Hampton S. Rearfoot posture in subjects with patellofemoral pain. *J Orthop Sports Phys Ther.* 1995; 22(4):155-160.

25. Reilly DT, Martens M. Experimental analysis of quadriceps muscle force and patellofemoral joint reaction force for various activities. *Acta Orthop Scand.* 1972; 43:126.

26. Fulkerson J, Hungerford DS. *Disorders of the Patellofemoral Joint.* 2nd ed. Baltimore, Md: Williams & Wilkins; 1990.

27. Flynn T, Soutas-Little R. Patellofemoral joint compressive forces in forward and backward walking. *J Ortho Sports Phys Ther.* 1995; 21(5):277-282.

28. Fu FH, Stone DA. Sports Injuries: *Mechanisms, Prevention and Treatment.* Baltimore, Md: Williams & Wilkins; 1994.

29. DeHaven KE. Rationale for meniscus repair or excision. *Clin Sports Med.* 1985; 4(2):267-274.

Suggested Reading

Arnoczky SD. The blood supply of the meniscus and its role in healing and repair. In: Finerman G, ed. *AAOS Symposium on Sports Medicine: The Knee.* St. Louis, Mo: CV Mosby; 1985.

Arnoczky SD, Warren RT. The microvasculature of the meniscus and its response to injury: An experimental study in the dog. *Am J Sports Med.* 1983; 11:131.

Basmajian J. Muscles Alive. Baltimore, Md: Williams & Wilkins; 1980.

Clancy WG, Shelbourne KD, Zoellner GB. Treatment of knee joint stability secondary to rupture of the posterior cruciate ligament: A report of a new procedure. *J Bone Joint Surg.* 1983; 65A:310.

Hay J, Reid J. *Anatomy, Mechanics and Human Motion.* Englewood Cliffs, NJ: Prentice Hall; 1988.

Hughston JC, Degenhait TC. Reconstruction of the posterior cruciate ligament. *Clin Orthop.* 1982; 164:59.

Kessler RM, Hertling D. *Management of Common Musculoskeletal Disorders: Physical Therapy Principles and Methods.* Philadelphia, Pa: JB Lippincott; 1993.

Knight RA. Developmental deformities of the lower extremities. *J Bone Joint Surg.* 1954; 36A:521.

McConnell J. The management of chondramalacia patellae: a long-term solution. *Australian Journal of Physical Therapy.* 1986; 32(4):214-223.

McCrea JD. *Pediatric Orthopaedics of the Lower Extremity.* New York, NY: Futura Publishing; 1985.

Rasch P. *Kinesiology and Applied Anatomy.* Philadelphia, Pa: Lea & Febiger; 1989.

Rodman GP, Schumacher HR. *Primer on the Rheumatic Diseases.* 8th ed. Antlanta, Ga: Arthritis Foundation; 1983.

Soderberg G. *Kinesiology: Application to Pathological Motion.* Baltimore, Md: Williams & Wilkins; 1986.

Stachli LT. Rotational problems of the lower extremities. *Orthop Clin North Am.* 1987; 18:503.

Torselli PA, Xianghia D, Warren RF. The effect of joint compressive load and quadriceps muscle force on knee motion in the intact and anterior cruciate ligament-sectioned knee. *Am J Sports Med.* 1994; 22(1):105-112.

1. Identify and palpate the bony prominence of the tibiofemoral and patellofemoral joints.

2. Explain the relationship between coxa vara and coxa valga of the hip to genu varum and genu valgum at the knee.

3. Explain the difference between a static and a dynamic Q-angle assessment.

4. Explain what happens to the patella when there is atrophy of the vastus medialis obliquus.

5. Why does a person who has undergone a patellectomy need special consideration during rehabilitation exercises?

6. Indicate how a meniscectomy affects joint surfaces.

7. Describe the screw home mechanism.

8. List the structures that predispose one to patellofemoral dysfunction.

9. Why would one choose to use open chain versus closed chain exercises for knee rehabilitation?

10. How does the angle of knee flexion affect patellofemoral joint reaction forces?

11. How does osteoarthritis develop? Is it preventable?

CHAPTER 12

THE ANKLE AND FOOT COMPLEX

Glenn P. Brown, MMSc, PT, ATC, SCS

OBJECTIVES

After completion of this chapter, the reader will be able to:

DIDACTIC

1. Identify relevant anatomical and functional units of the ankle and foot.
2. Define triplane motion and give examples of its relevance to the major joints of the foot.
3. Identify the locations and functions of the ligaments of the ankle and foot.
4. Describe the muscular function of the foot during each phase of gait.
5. Identify biomechanical implications for injury to the major musculotendinous structures of the ankle and foot complex.
6. Identify factors that contribute to abnormal pronation and supination of the foot and the effects of each.

PRACTICAL

1. Palpate relevant anatomical landmarks of the ankle and foot.
2. Demonstrate the difference between open and closed chain pronation and supination.
3. Demonstrate the normal sequence of pronation and supination in the foot during the phases of gait.
4. Demonstrate the windlass effect of the plantar fascia.
5. Assess the torque conversion that occurs at the subtalar joint.
6. Assess normal and abnormal pronation and supination of the foot.
7. Recognize the stresses needed to disrupt normal ligamentous integrity of the ankle and foot.

ANATOMICAL CONSIDERATIONS

The foot is comprised of 28 bones, at least 29 bony articulations, and a great number of supporting ligaments.[1] Functionally, the foot is divided into an upper and lower unit. The upper functional unit is comprised of the talus and lower leg. The lower functional unit includes the calcaneus and the rest of the foot. The foot is also further divided into forefoot, midfoot, and rearfoot components.[2] The rearfoot consists of the talus and calcaneus, while the midfoot contains the navicular, cuboid, and cuneiform bones. The forefoot is comprised of the metatarsals and phalanges. As a whole, the ankle and foot together serve four main functions:

1. Serve as a base of support
2. Act as a shock absorber
3. Act as a mobile adapter
4. Serve as a rigid lever

OSTEOLOGY

The distal ends of both the tibia and fibula form the superior aspect of the ankle. The bones of the ankle and foot can be seen in Figure 12-1. Each bone has multiple articulations that lead to the complexity of joint movement within the foot. The bones in the foot are referred to as tarsals and include the calcaneus, talus, navicular, cuboid, and three cuneiforms. Distal to the tarsals are metatarsals, and then the phalanges. Each metatarsal and phalange, like the metacarpals and phalanges in the hand, contain a base (proximal), a shaft (middle), and a head (distal).

The foot contains two arches: the longitudinal arch and transverse arch. These are soft tissue structures that provide support to the bony articulations and configurations. The longitudinal arch (Figure 12-2) is described as an arc based posteriorly at the calcaneus and anteriorly at the metatarsal heads. The arch is continuous both medially and laterally through the foot. Because the longitudinal arch is higher medially, it is usually the side of reference.[3]

The transverse arch is also a continuous structure, being most prominent at the level of the anterior tarsals and gradually becoming less concave distally and nearly flat at the level of the metatarsal heads (Figures 12-3a and 12-3b). In some instances, one of the metatarsal heads may be plantarflexed. When this condition occurs, the

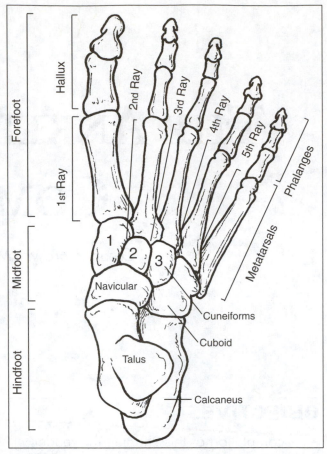

Figure 12-1. A schematic diagram of the bones and subdivisions of the foot.

plantarflexed metatarsal incurs greater ground reaction forces and is more susceptible to repetitive stress injuries, such as metatarsalgia and stress fractures. The first metatarsal is the most common sight for this condition to occur, but it can occur in the second or third, giving the transverse arch a more convex appearance. Because the first metatarsal is more dense and better designed to withstand forces than the other metatarsals, it is better able to withstand these additional stresses, as seen with a plantarflexed condition. When the second or third metatarsals are plantarflexed and are forced to accept a greater weightbearing load, they take on a greater risk of injury.

MUSCULAR ANATOMY

Muscles that act on the ankle and foot are referred to as either intrinsic or extrinsic. Similar to muscles of the hand and wrist, those muscles that originate and insert within the foot itself are referred to as intrinsic. Those that originate proxi-

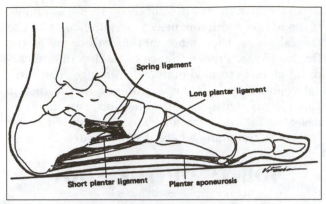

Figure 12-2. The medial longitudinal arch of the foot with its associated ligamentous support (the plantar ligaments are projected through from the lateral side of the foot) (reprinted with permission from Norkin CN, Levangie PK. *Joint Structure and Function: A Comprehensive Analysis*. Philadelphia, Pa: FA Davis; 1983).

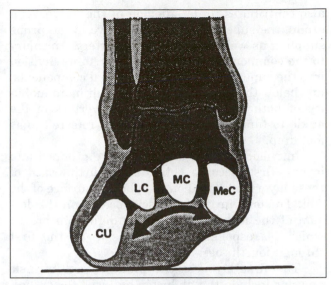

Figure 12-3a. The transverse arch at the level of anterior tarsals. (Cu = cuboid; LC = lateral cuneiform; MC = middle cuneiform; MeC = medial cuneiform) (reprinted with permission from Norkin CN, Levangie PK. *Joint Structure and Function: A Comprehensive Analysis*. Philadelphia, Pa: FA Davis; 1983).

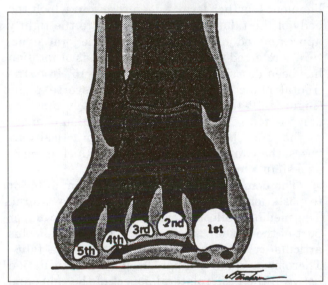

Figure 12-3b. The transverse arch at the level of the metatarsals (reprinted with permission from Norkin CN, Levangie PK. *Joint Structure and Function: A Comprehensive Analysis*. Philadelphia, Pa: FA Davis; 1983).

mal to the ankle joint, cross the ankle, and then insert into the foot are considered extrinsic muscles.

The extrinsic muscles of the lower leg and ankle are classified most commonly by compartments. There are four compartments: anterior, posterior, deep posterior, and lateral. Anterior compartment muscles may also be called pretibial muscles. Muscles included in this compartment are the tibialis anterior, extensor hallucis longus, and extensor digitorum longus. As a group, these muscles are innervated by the deep peroneal nerve,

while the anterior tibial artery supplies blood to this region. The primary action of anterior compartment muscles is to dorsiflex the ankle concentrically and control the lowering plantarflexion of the ankle eccentrically.

Muscles of the posterior compartment include the gastrocnemius, soleus, and plantaris. Together, these three muscles are referred to as the triceps surae. The gastrocnemius and soleus are primarily powerful plantarflexors, while the plantaris contributes little to function, as it is a very long and thin muscle almost tendon-like throughout its entire length. Muscles of the posterior compartment receive neural innervation from the tibial nerve and blood supply from the posterior tibial artery.

The deep posterior compartment muscles are the flexor hallucis longus, the flexor digitorum longus, and the tibialis posterior. These muscles are also innervated by the tibial nerve and receive blood supply from the posterior tibial artery. Since each muscle crosses the ankle joint and is located posteriorly, they will contribute to plantarflexion of the ankle. However, the major action of the flexor hallucis longus and the flexor digitorum longus is to perform flexion of the great toe and the lateral four digits, respectively.

The lateral compartment contains the muscles most responsible for performing eversion of the ankle. These muscles consist of the peroneal longus, brevis, and tertius. The peroneus tertius also contributes to dorsiflexion of the ankle. As a group, the superficial peroneal nerve is the prime supplier, as well as the peroneal artery. An injury to the common peroneal nerve prior to its division into the superficial and deep peroneal components, just below the fibular head, will result in an inability of both the dorsiflexors and evertors of the ankle to function. This condition is referred to as foot drop.

Intrinsic muscles of the foot are grouped into layers: first, second, third, and fourth. Each of these layers is located on the plantar surface of the foot. The only intrinsic muscle located on the dorsum of the foot is the extensor digitorum brevis, which is responsible for extension of the first through fourth toes.

The first layer of the plantar foot intrinsic muscles include the abductor hallucis, flexor digitorum brevis, and abductor digiti minimi. While each contributes to movement of the toes (see Appendix A), they also serve to assist with the stability of the arches in the feet. The second layer includes the quadratus plantae and the lumbricales. The third layer is made up of the flexor hallucis brevis, adductor hallucis, and flexor digiti minimi. The fourth layer includes both the dorsal and plantar interossei muscles.

ARTHROKINEMATICS OF THE ANKLE AND FOOT

Triplane motion is a motion that takes place in all three body planes due to an axis of motion that makes an angle with all three planes. This is much different than singular plane motion, which has been discussed in great detail up to this point. Triplane motion is formed in the foot as a result of a combination of singular plane motions as described:

- Frontal plane: inversion and eversion
- Sagittal plane: dorsiflexion and plantarflexion
- Transverse plane: abduction and adduction

The major joints of the foot have axes that make an angle with these three cardinal planes and therefore exhibit triplane motion. The most commonly referred to triplane movements in the foot are pronation and supination. Pronation is a combined movement of dorsiflexion, abduction, and eversion. By contrast, supination is a combination of plantarflexion, adduction, and inversion. The amount of motion occurring in each body plane depends upon the position of the axis. For example, if the axis of motion is nearly perpendicular to the frontal plane, then more motion will occur in the frontal plane. Predominance of motion in one cardinal plane is termed planar dominance. The clinical relevance of planar dominance in the foot is that joints with triplane motion can best be assessed for their motion capability by observing motion in the plane where it most occurs.

JOINTS OF THE FOOT

Talocrural Joint

The ankle or talocrural joint is a uni-axial joint. The lower fibula and its malleolus, the lower tibia and its malleolus, and the inferior transverse ligament together form a deep recess in which the body of the talus is embraced.[1] Due to the tightly approximated joint surfaces, the ankle joint structure is referred to as a mortise. The axis of rotation has been described as being oriented 15° from the frontal plane and 8° from the transverse plane (Figures 12-4a and 12-4b). However, it must be emphasized that the true axis of rotation changes as the joint changes positions. For practical purposes, the joint can be considered to function more as a simple hinge joint.

The dome of the talus is convex from anterior to posterior and concave from medial to lateral. The medial malleolus articulates with the upper part of the medial talus, and the lateral malleolus articulates with the lateral aspect of the talus. There is a small triangular shaped articulation between the posterolateral aspect of the talus and the inferior transverse ligament. The articular surfaces of the ankle mortise are the most congruent in the body.[4]

The integrity of the ankle mortise is dependent upon the solid union of the tibia and fibula. The union is maintained by two joints that are anatomically distinct from the ankle joint but function to serve the ankle. These two joints are the superior and inferior tibiofibular joints. The superior tibiofibular joint is a plane synovial joint formed by the head of the fibula and the posterolateral aspect of the tibia and surrounded by a joint capsule that is reinforced by anterior and posterior ligaments. The motions that occur at this joint are superior and inferior gliding of the fibula, as well as fibular rotation.

The inferior tibiofibular joint is a syndesmosis,

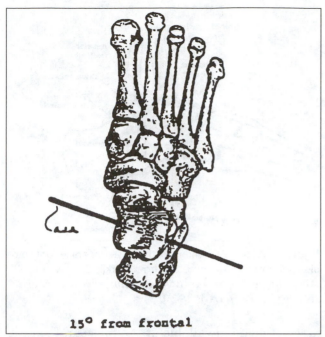

15° from frontal

Figure 12-4a. The orientation of the ankle joint axis of motion from the frontal plane (reprinted with permission from Root ML, Orien WP, Weed JH. *Clinical Biomechanics. Vol II: Normal and Abnormal Function of the Foot.* Los Angeles, Calif: Clinical Biomechanics Corporation; 1977).

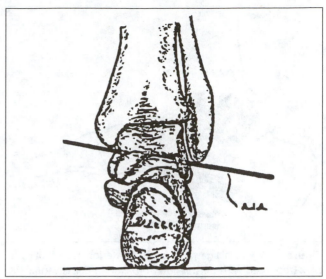

Figure 12-4b. The orientation of the ankle joint axis of motion from the transverse plane (reprinted with permission from Root ML, Orien WP, Weed JH. *Clinical Biomechanics. Vol II: Normal and Abnormal Function of the Foot.* Los Angeles, Calif: Clinical Biomechanics Corporation; 1977).

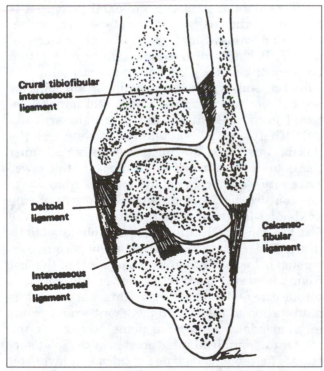

Figure 12-5. Ligaments of the subtalar joint (cross section, posterior view) (reprinted with permission from Norkin CN, Levangie PK. *Joint Structure and Function: A Comprehensive Analysis.* Philadelphia, Pa: FA Davis; 1983).

or fibrous union, between the concave facet of the distal tibia and the convex facet of the distal fibula. The two bones are separated by fibrocartilaginous tissue. There is no joint capsule since it is not a synovial joint. However, there are several important ligaments. The most important of these is the crural tibiofibular interosseous ligament (Figure 12-5). Its oblique fibers run for a short distance between the distal tibia and fibula, maintaining the joint integrity. The ligament is so strong that stresses forcing the two bones apart will often result in a fracture of the distal fibula before disruption of the ligament occurs. The other ligaments that support the inferior tibiofibular joint are the anterior and posterior tibiofibular ligaments and the interosseous membrane. These ligaments are significantly weaker than the crural tibiofibular interosseous ligament.

LIGAMENTS OF THE TALOCRURAL JOINT

The talocrural joint depends upon a fully intact ligamentous structure for normal stability because the joint capsule is thin and weak, particularly anteriorly to posteriorly. The medial ligament complex is made up of the strong deltoid ligament (Figure 12-6). The deltoid ligament is fan-shaped and arises from the borders of the medial malleolus and attaches in a continuous line on the navicular anteriorly and the talus and calcaneus posteriorly and distally. Forces that would often gap the medial side of the joint will often result in an avul-

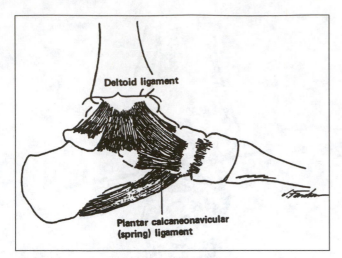

Figure 12-6. Medial ligaments of the posterior ankle-foot complex (reprinted with permission from Norkin CN, Levangie PK. *Joint Structure and Function: A Comprehensive Analysis.* Philadelphia, Pa: FA Davis; 1983).

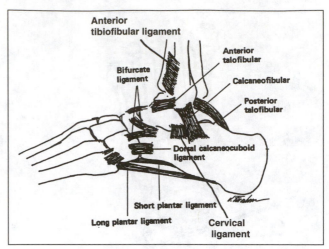

Figure 12-7. Lateral ligaments of the posterior ankle-foot complex (reprinted with permission from Norkin CN, Levangie PK. *Joint Structure and Function: A Comprehensive Analysis.* Philadelphia, Pa: FA Davis; 1983).

sion fracture of the medial malleolus rather than a disruption of the ligament itself as a result of its strength. However, sprains to the deltoid ligament can occur and are seen in roughly 15% to 20% of all ankle ligament sprains.

The lateral ligament complex is comprised of (from anterior to posterior) the anterior talofibular ligament, the calcaneofibular ligament, and the posterior talofibular ligament (Figure 12-7). The anterior talofibular ligament is actually a capsular ligament reinforcing the anterolateral capsule over the sinus tarsi region. The attachments of the lateral ligaments are evident by their names. These lateral ligaments resist gapping of the lateral side of the ankle joint and are injured more frequently than the deltoid ligament. Sprains of the lateral ankle ligaments are most commonly seen as a result of an inversion twisting mechanism while the foot is planted on the ground.

TALOCRURAL JOINT OSTEOKINEMATICS

Because the ankle joint axis is nearly perpendicular to the sagittal plane, the dominant motion is dorsiflexion/plantarflexion. There are small components of abduction/adduction and inversion/eversion but these are clinically insignificant. During dorsiflexion, the wider anterior portion of the talar articular surface requires widening of the tibiofibular syndesmosis. This is accomplished by a slight lateral rotation of the fibula.[1] The talar dome, which is convex anterior to posterior, exhibits a posterior glide of the talus on the tibiofibular mortise during dorsiflexion. The converse is true during plantarflexion. The normal range of motion available at the talocrural joint is approximately 20° of dorsiflexion and between 30° and 50° of plantarflexion.

Subtalar Joint

The subtalar joint is a uni-axial joint that is formed by the articulations between the calcaneus and talus. Since it has a single axis of motion, it has 1° of freedom. Due to its location between the ankle joint and midtarsal joint, the subtalar joint is an extremely important joint for normal foot function. The upper and lower functional units meet at the subtalar joint articulation. Therefore, the subtalar joint serves as the link between the two functional units and must serve to convert rotatory torques in the lower extremity.[5] Transverse plane motions from above are converted into frontal plane motions in the ankle and foot, and frontal plane motions in the foot are converted into transverse plane motions in the lower leg. The mechanism of torque conversion is essential to protect the joints of the foot from potentially destructive forces. Without this torque conversion mechanism, internal and external rotation of the tibia during gait would result in tremendous transverse plane torques at the talocrural joint, leading to erosion of the joint surfaces. The same holds true for calcaneal inversion and eversion, which would result in frontal plane torques at the talocrural joint and eventually erode the articular surfaces.

The subtalar joint is comprised of two articular areas, located anteriorly and posteriorly. The

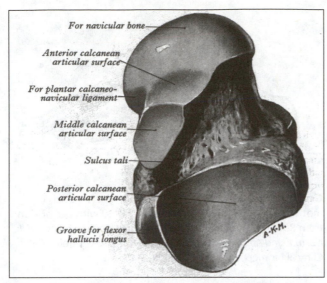

Figure 12-8a. The plantar/inferior aspect of the left talus (reprinted with permission from Williams PL, Warwick R, Dyson M, Banniste LH. *Gray's Anatomy*. 37th ed. London: Churchill Livingstone; 1989).

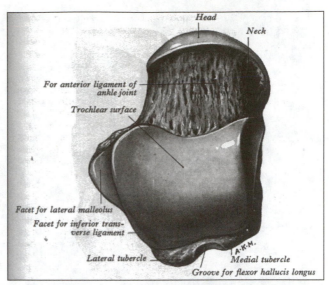

Figure 12-8b. The dorsal aspect of the left calcaneus (reprinted with permission from Williams PL, Warwick R, Dyson M, Banniste LH. *Gray's Anatomy*. 37th ed. London: Churchill Livingstone; 1989).

largest articular surface is the posterior articulation, which is comprised of the posterior convex calcaneal facet and the reciprocal posterior concave facet of the talus. Between the posterior and anterior articulations, there is a bony tunnel formed by the grooves on the inferior talus (sulcus tali) and the superior calcaneus (sulcus calcanei). The tunnel is referred to as the tarsal canal and opens superolaterally to the sinus tarsi (Figures 12-8a and 12-8b). The anterior articulation is more variable and consists of two or three articulating facets. The calcaneal facets lie on the sustentaculum tali, which serves to support and provide articulation with the reciprocating facets on the inferior surface of the talar body and neck. The anterior articulation shares its joint capsule with the talonavicular portion of the midtarsal joint. These two joints—the subtalar and the midtarsal—function intimately together.

LIGAMENTS OF THE SUBTALAR JOINT

The most significant ligament that directly supports the subtalar joint is the interosseous talocalcaneal ligament (see Figure 12-5). The interosseous talocalcaneal ligament is located in the tarsal canal and runs obliquely downward and laterally from the talar sulcus to the calcaneal sulcus. The ligament is most taut with eversion of the calcaneus. The cervical ligament is just lateral to the sinus tarsi and attached to the upper surface of the calcaneus and passes upward and medially to a tubercle on the inferior and lateral aspects of the

talus. The cervical ligament is taut when the foot is inverted. In addition to the interosseous talocalcaneal ligament and the cervical ligament, the subtalar joint receives direct support from the medial and lateral ankle ligaments and indirect support from the ligaments of the midtarsal joint.

SUBTALAR JOINT OSTEOKINEMATICS

Pronation and supination are the motions present in the subtalar joint. The average subtalar joint axis is oriented 42° from the horizontal plane and 16° from the sagittal plane[5-7] (Figures 12-9a and 12-9b). Therefore, the dominant planes of motion are the frontal (inversion/eversion) and transverse (abduction/adduction). Minimal sagittal plane motion is present at the subtalar joint due to the axis not being oriented in a predominantly medial/lateral direction. The orientation of the axis varies among individuals and will affect the planar dominance of motion. For example, the vertical orientation of the subtalar joint axis may vary from 20° to 60° from the transverse plane. The effect of this variation is that the planar dominance will be more in the transverse plane when the axis is more vertical and more in the frontal plane when the axis has a lower inclination. The clinical relevance of this is that individuals with lower inclination angles will have greater stresses in the foot compared to more stresses being transferred up the kinetic chain.

In an open kinetic chain, the calcaneus moves on the talus. However, the ground reaction forces

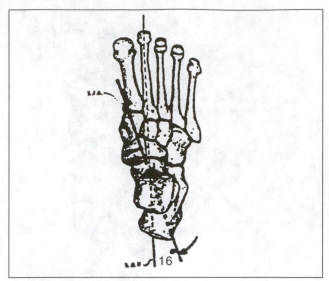

Figure 12-9a. The orientation of the subtalar joint axis of motion from the sagittal plane (reprinted with permission from Root ML, Orien WP, Weed JH. *Clinical Biomechanics. Vol II: Normal and Abnormal Function of the Foot.* Los Angeles, Calif: Clinical Biomechanics Corporation; 1977).

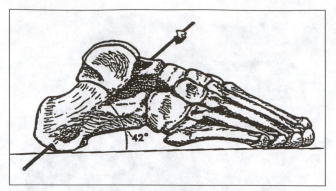

Figure 12-9b. The orientation of the subtalar joint axis of motion form the transverse plane (reprinted with permission from Root ML, Orien WP, Weed JH. *Clinical Biomechanics. Vol II: Normal and Abnormal Function of the Foot.* Los Angeles, Calif: Clinical Biomechanics Corporation; 1977).

associated with weightbearing limit the calcaneus from moving in the transverse and sagittal planes during gait. In the closed kinetic chain, pronation is accomplished by eversion (frontal plane) and adduction (transverse plane) of the calcaneus and slight plantarflexion (sagittal plane) of the talus. In the same way, closed chain supination consists of calcaneal inversion (frontal plane) and abduction (transverse plane), as well as dorsiflexion (sagittal plane) of the talus.

The Midtarsal Joint

The midtarsal joint is an S-shaped joint comprised of the articulation between the talus and navicular on the medial side and the calcaneus and the cuboid on the lateral side (Figure 12-10). The joint has two axes of motion: an oblique axis and a longitudinal axis. Due to its proximity to the subtalar joint, the two joints cannot function independently from one another. Motion at the subtalar joint must result in changes of position at the midtarsal joint due to the talar articulation with the navicular and the sharing of a joint capsule. The proper function of these two joints working together with the talocrural joint is critical for normal foot mechanics.

The talonavicular articulation has been likened to the hip joint in that it approximates a ball and socket articulation. By contrast, the calcaneocuboid articulation is saddle-shaped and is

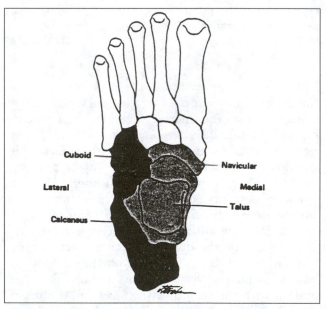

Figure 12-10. The talonavicular joint and calcaneocuboid joint from a compound, S-shaped joint line that transects the foot. They are collectively referred to as the midtarsal joint (reprinted with permission from Norkin CN, Levangie PK. *Joint Structure and Function: A Comprehensive Analysis.* Philadelphia, Pa: FA Davis; 1983).

therefore more restrictive in mobility versus the talonavicular articulation.

LIGAMENTS OF THE MIDTARSAL JOINT

The plantar surface of the talonavicular articulation is formed by the plantar calcaneonavicular (spring) ligament (see Figure 12-2). The spring ligament is a triangular sheet arising from the sustentaculum tali and attaching to the inferior surface of the navicular. Its central portion supports the talar head and is covered with fibrocartilage.[3]

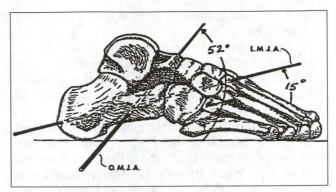

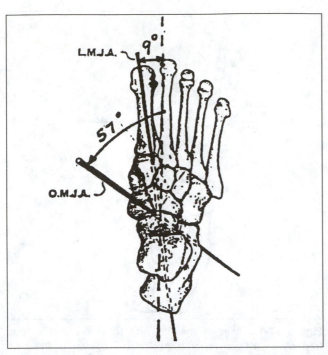

Figure 12-11a. The orientation of the midtarsal joint axes of motion from the sagittal plane (OMJA = oblique midtarsal joint axis; LMJA = longitudinal midtarsal joint axis) (reprinted with permission from Root ML, Orien WP, Weed JH. *Clinical Biomechanics. Vol II: Normal and Abnormal Function of the Foot.* Los Angeles, Calif: Clinical Biomechanics Corporation; 1977).

Figure 12-11b. The orientation of the midtarsal joint axes of motion from the transverse plane (OMJA = oblique midtarsal joint axis; LMJA = longitudinal midtarsal joint axis) (reprinted with permission from Root ML, Orien WP, Weed JH. *Clinical Biomechanics. Vol II: Normal and Abnormal Function of the Foot.* Los Angeles, Calif: Clinical Biomechanics Corporation; 1977).

The spring ligament is continuous medially with the superficial portion of the deltoid ligament.[1,3] It functions to deepen the articular cavity of the talonavicular joint and limit flattening of the medial longitudinal arch. The bifurcate ligament has two bands, as its name suggests (see Figure 12-7). The medial or calcaneonavicular band attaches from the anterior and dorsal calcaneus to the dorsolateral part of the navicular. The lateral or calcaneocuboid band attaches to the medial aspect of the cuboid, arising from the same location as the calcaneonavicular band. The bifurcate ligament resists adduction and plantarflexion of the midtarsal joint. It is often injured along with the lateral ligaments of the ankle as a result of an inversion type sprain.

Also supporting the calcaneonavicular ligament are the long and short plantar ligaments (see Figure 12-7). The long plantar ligament is the longest of the tarsal ligaments and attaches posteriorly from the plantar surface of the calcaneus near the medial tuberosity and continues forward to the base of the second, third, and fourth metatarsals. The long plantar ligament has great tensile strength and limits flattening of the lateral longitudinal arch. This ligament also converts the

groove on the plantar surface of the cuboid into a tunnel for the peroneal longus tendon. The short plantar ligament is a short, but wide, band of great strength. It stretches from the anterior tubercle of the calcaneus to the adjoining part of the plantar surface of the cuboid bone and also functions to limit flattening of the lateral longitudinal arch.

MIDTARSAL JOINT OSTEOKINEMATICS

As mentioned, the midtarsal joint has two axes of motion referred to as the longitudinal axis and the oblique axis, thus demonstrating 2 of freedom. The oblique axis is oriented 52 from the horizontal and 57 from the sagittal plane[5] (Figures 12-11a and 12-11b). Due to the orientation of the oblique axis, very little motion is present in the frontal plane. By contrast, much motion is present in the transverse plane and the sagittal plane. The predominant movements are abduction/adduction in the transverse plane and dorsiflexion and plantarflexion in the sagittal plane. One clinical note of significance relates to the availability of dorsiflexion at the oblique midtarsal joint axis. When a person exhibits insufficient ankle joint dorsiflexion (less than 10 with the knee extended) during gait, additional dorsiflexion may be obtained at the midtarsal joint along the oblique axis. Although additional dorsiflexion is an apparently good response from the midtarsal joint, the mechanical cost to the foot may outweigh the benefits because it can lead to abnormal and excessive pronation.

The longitudinal axis, as its name implies, has nearly a straight anterior-posterior orientation. The axis is oriented just 15 from the transverse plane and only 9 from the sagittal plane[5] (see Figures 12-11a and 12-11b). The predominant motion occurring here is frontal plane inversion and eversion.

As mentioned previously, a close interrelationship exists between the subtalar and midtarsal joints. The midtarsal joint is free to move when the subtalar joint is pronated. When the subtalar joint is supinated, however, it becomes locked and exhibits a significant decrease in available motion. This locking and unlocking of the midtarsal joint becomes very important when the foot functions during gait. When this mechanism is functioning well, the foot functions well as both a shock absorber and mobile adapter to uneven terrain during the contact and midstance portions of gait, and also as a rigid lever for propulsion at toe-off. Much of the biomechanical pathology of the foot is related to disruption of this mechanism.

Tarsometatarsal Joint

The tarsometatarsal joint (TMT) is actually a series of plane synovial articulations formed by the distal tarsal row and the bases of the metatarsals. The first TMT joint is formed by the articulation between the base of the first metatarsal and the medial cuneiform, and actually has its own joint capsule. The second TMT joint consists of a mortise formed by the middle cuneiform and the sides of the medial and lateral cuneiforms, which articulate with the base of the second metatarsal. This joint is the strongest and least mobile of the TMT joints and is also set slightly more posterior than the others. The third TMT joint is formed by the third metatarsal and lateral cuneiform. It shares a capsule with the second TMT joint. The fourth and fifth TMT joints are formed by the bases of the fourth and fifth metatarsals and the cuboid. These two articulations also share a joint capsule. Furthermore, small plane articulations exist between the bases of the metatarsals, which permit small amounts of gliding motion between the metatarsals themselves.

TARSOMETATARSAL JOINT OSTEOKINEMATICS

Each TMT joint is considered to have its own axis of motion.[5] Each metatarsal and its associated cuneiform (first through third) or the metatarsal itself (fourth and fifth) are termed rays. The first ray is the most mobile, followed by the fifth ray. The axis of motion of the first and fifth rays converge and are oblique and therefore triplanar (Figure 12-12). The fifth ray axis is oriented from posterior, inferior, and lateral as it then travels toward an anterior, superior, and medial direction;

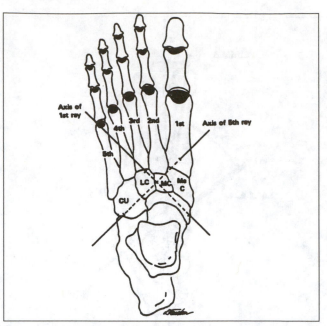

Figure 12-12. Axes of the first and fifth rays of the foot (reprinted with permission from Norkin CN, Levangie PK. *Joint Structure and Function: A Comprehensive Analysis*. Philadelphia, Pa: FA Davis; 1983).

therefore, motions occurring here are primarily pronation and supination. The first ray axis is different in that it is oriented from posterior, inferior, and medial to an anterior, superior, and lateral direction. The motion at the first ray is also triplanar but is not described as pronation and supination. Rather, the combined movements are:
1. dorsiflexion, adduction, and inversion
2. plantarflexion, abduction, and eversion

The TMT joint functions to regulate the position of the metatarsal heads and phalanges relative to weightbearing surfaces. For example, when the rearfoot everts, the TMT will invert to counter rotate the foot. This counter rotation requires the first ray to dorsiflex and the fifth ray to plantarflex in order to maintain a more even weight distribution on the metatarsal heads and phalanges. The opposite is seen when the hindfoot is inverted; however, the ability to move is somewhat restricted as a result of the osseous stability, or locking, that occurs when the subtalar joint is supinated. Since the first and fifth rays are the most mobile, the greatest amount of compensation occurs at these two rays.

Metatarsalphalangeal Joint

The metatarsophalangeal (MTP) joints are condyloid joints with 2 of freedom: flexion/extension and abduction/adduction. These joints are formed by the concave articular surface of the proximal phalanx of each toe and the corresponding convex metatarsal head. The primary function of the MTP joints is to allow the foot to pass over the toes during gait. This function involves extension of the toes at the MTP joint and also consists of two other mechanisms, referred to as the metatarsal break and the windlass effect.

The metatarsal break refers to the oblique angle of the metatarsal heads, which contribute to lateral transferring of body weight as one approaches toe-off.[8] The lateral transfer of weight occurs in the terminal portions of the stance phase, as one's body weight is then transferred to the forefoot. The lateral transfer of body weight causes the calcaneus to invert and can therefore contribute to subtalar joint supination. The windlass effect refers to the tensing of the plantar fascia by the extension of the MTP joints during the terminal stance phase of gait. Tensing results from the attachment of the plantar fascia into the proximal phalanx of the toes. As the plantar fascia becomes tense, it causes the arch to rise, thus the subtalar joint supinates. This allows for assistance of the foot to become a rigid lever for propulsion.

Interphalangeal Joint

The interphalangeal joints of the toes are synovial hinge joints that possess 1° of freedom: flexion and extension. There are five proximal interphalangeal (PIP) joints and four distal interphalangeal (DIP) joints. Each is nearly identical in structure to its counterpart in the hand. The toes function primarily to help maintain stability by pressing against the ground both in static posture and during gait.

FOOT FUNCTION DURING GAIT

The gait cycle can be broken down into two phases: the stance phase and the swing phase. The stance phase can be further divided into three phases: contact, midstance, and propulsive phases.[6] The contact phase begins when the heel strikes the ground and continues until the toe-off of the opposite foot. The stance foot is now flat on the walking surface. The midstance phase begins at the point in which the foot is flat on the walking surface and ends with heel lift. The propulsive phase represents the final portion of the stance

phase and ends when the toes come off of the walking surface. A more indepth look at the gait cycle, as well as a further explanation of the various terms used to describe the phases of gait, can be found in Chapter 13.

The Contact Phase

JOINT FUNCTION

As mentioned, the contact phase begins when the heel hits the walking surface. During this time, the calcaneus typically strikes the ground in a slightly inverted position, indicating that the subtalar joint is slightly supinated.[9] The calcaneus everts approximately 4° to 6° immediately after hitting the ground, resulting in subtalar joint pronation that assists in the shock-absorbing process that is necessary at initial contact. Subtalar joint pronation unlocks the midtarsal joint so that when the foot hits the ground, it is a more supple structure that is capable of adapting to uneven terrain. The lower leg internally rotates as it follows the adduction of the talus via the ankle mortise. Thus, the frontal plane motion of calcaneal eversion is converted into the transverse plane motion of internal rotation by the subtalar joint.

The ankle joint moves rapidly into plantarflexion as the foot becomes flat on the floor. The body center of pressure is located on the lateral side of the foot. The ground reaction force on the lateral side assists in the pronation that occurs during the contact phase.[6]

MUSCLE FUNCTION

The predominant muscle function during the contact phase is eccentric control of deceleration. The anterior compartment muscles function to decelerate the rapid plantar flexion of the ankle. In addition, the tibialis anterior functions to decelerate the rapid pronation that is occurring. This is accomplished since the tibialis anterior has a muscular attachment medial to the subtalar joint axis. The gastrocnemius and the soleus also function to decelerate pronation and internal rotation of the lower leg in the late contact phase.

Midstance Phase

JOINT FUNCTION

During midstance, the foot is converted from being a mobile adapter to a rigid lever for propulsion. The subtalar joint begins to supinate from the maximally pronated position. Supination is the result of a combined effort by the supinating muscles of the foot and the external rotation of the leg that results from pelvic rotation. The transverse plane motion of external rotation is converted into the frontal plane motion of calcaneal eversion via supination of the subtalar joint. By late midstance, just prior to heel-off, the subtalar joint reaches its neutral position where it is neither pronated nor supinated. With the subtalar joint near neutral, the foot is now prepared to become a rigid lever for propulsion due to the locking effect that the subtalar joint has on the rest of the foot. The ankle joint moves from a position of plantarflexion to approximately 10° of dorsiflexion by late midstance, just prior to heel-off. The body's center of pressure begins to move medially so that most of the pressure is centralized just lateral and proximal to the first metatarsal head.[6]

MUSCLE FUNCTION

The soleus, posterior tibialis, flexor digitorum longus, and flexor hallucis longus function to decelerate the forward movement of the tibia as it progresses over the foot to increase dorsiflexion. The forces generated by these four muscles would contribute to hyperextension of the knee if it were not for the antagonistic function of the gastrocnemius, which exerts a knee flexion force that stabilizes the knee from hyperextending. The posterior tibialis and the gastrocnemius/soleus complex also function to assist in supinating the subtalar joint.

Propulsive Phase

JOINT FUNCTION

Supination continues at the subtalar joint to further enhance the skeletal efficiency of the foot to function as a rigid lever for propulsion. The lower leg continues to externally rotate and the ankle joint plantarflexes rapidly from its position of 10° of dorsiflexion to 20° of plantarflexion as the foot pushes off the ground.[10] The toes begin to bear weight during the propulsive phase. The MTP joints move into extension as the ankle plantarflexes. Sixty-five degrees of extension are required at the first MTP to allow the foot to progress over the hallux at toe-off. The metatarsal break also contributes to the supination that occurs during the propulsive phase. Despite the lateral weight-shifting effect of the metatarsal break, the body's net center of pressure remains over the first metatarsal and hallux.

MUSCLE FUNCTION

The gastrocnemius and soleus function to assist heel-off during early propulsion. The gastrocnemius does this by flexing the knee and soleus by decelerating the forward momentum of the tibia, thus resulting in "pulling" the heel off the ground. The peroneus longus functions to stabilize the first ray against the ground, thereby preventing it from moving into dorsiflexion as the body weight moves over the first ray. If the first ray was to dorsiflex, the foot would compensate by rolling over into pronation at a time when the foot needs to be supinated.

The abductor hallucis, flexor hallucis brevis, extensor hallucis brevis, and adductor hallucis function to stabilize the first MTP during toe-off. The intrinsic muscles in the arch function to assist in stabilizing the arch structure during propulsion. The peroneus longus and brevis function antagonistically to the supination that is occurring during propulsion to balance out these forces and add further stability.

BIOMECHANICAL FACTORS ASSOCIATED WITH COMMON INJURIES

Many overuse injuries to the ankle and foot complex, as well as the entire lower quarter, can be attributed to abnormal mechanics. Overuse injuries can be precipitated or perpetuated by abnormal biomechanics. Most commonly, abnormal biomechanics occur as a result of the foot compensating for structural or soft tissue abnormalities.[6] Abnormal pronation is the most common form of compensation since the flattening of the arch and plantarflexion of the talus are assisted by gravity, whereas abnormal supination requires more energy to raise the arch and lift the talus into dorsiflexion.

Abnormal Pronation

There are two ways in which pronation can be considered abnormal. Subtalar joint pronation can be:

- excessive in terms of the amount of pronation
- abnormal due to the subtalar joint being pronated when it should be supinated

From a clinical perspective, it is easy to identify an excessively pronated foot by observing a very flattened arch and everted calcaneus. However, identification of abnormal timing of pronation requires a firm knowledge of the normal sequences of pronation and supination during gait.

The adverse effects of an abnormally pronated foot are a result of soft tissue structures having to provide greater stabilization and support to the joints of the foot. The additional stabilization demands are of greater consequence when the foot is pronated late in the midstance phase and into the propulsive phase. As mentioned earlier, the foot should be a rigid lever for propulsion. If it is pronated during the propulsive phase, additional support is required either from increased muscular stabilization or increased loads placed on the ligamentous and capsular structures. Over time, these increased demands can result in muscular or ligamentous overuse injuries. Ligamentous and capsular laxity may also result over time and can lead to subluxation of the joints of the foot, most notably the talonavicular articulation with the first MTP. This condition is called a hallux valgus deformity.

PATHOLOGIES ASSOCIATED WITH ABNORMAL PRONATION

When the foot pronates excessively during the contact phase of gait, then the tibialis anterior and posterior are placed under greater demand to decelerate subtalar joint pronation. The medial aspect of the achilles tendon is placed under greater tensile load due to the increased eversion of the calcaneus from the subtalar neutral position. The arch will flatten more than expected and the plantar fascia and spring ligament will undergo increased loading. Therefore, excessive pronation during the contact phase of gait can lead to breakdown of any of these structures. If the foot recovers from this excessive pronation later in the stance phase, then clinical manifestation of injuries to these musculotendinous and ligamentous structures are infrequent. The most common deformity that contributes to abnormal pronation in the contact phase is rearfoot varus, defined as an inversion deformity of the calcaneus when the subtalar joint is in its neutral position.[6] In order for the plantar surface of the calcaneus to be in contact with the ground, it must evert and therefore cause subtalar joint pronation.

When the foot is pronated excessively or is pronating later than normal during the midstance phase, the posterior tibialis is particularly vulnerable to injury due to its function to stabilize the arch by decelerating or limiting pronation. Additional load is placed on the posterior tibialis from ankle dorsiflexion that is occurring since it is also responsible for decelerating dorsiflexion. The combined demand of both functions can result in injury to the posterior tibialis tendon near the medial malleolus or at its attachment site. Injury to the tibial attachment is one cause of posteromedial shin splints, a common overuse injury in sports with high running demands.

The plantar fascia and spring ligament are also at risk due to the sustained flattening of the arch. The medial achilles tendon is vulnerable due to the combined tensile load of calcaneal eversion and ankle dorsiflexion. The gastrocnemius and soleus function to decelerate ankle dorsiflexion and also calcaneal eversion due to the quarter turn that is seen in the tendon, placing the soleus slightly more medial. The preferential tensile loading of the soleus can result in injury at its posterior tibial attachment and is another possible cause for posteromedial shin splints. The most common deformities that result in pronation late in the midstance phase are forefoot varus and tibial varum.

As previously discussed, if pronation continues into the propulsive phase of gait, it may lead to a higher than normal tensile force applied to the ligamentous and musculotendinous structures. The plantar fascia is particularly at risk when this occurs due to the combined effect of tension from flattening of the arch and from toe extension that occurs at the beginning of the windlass effect. With time, plantar fasciitis, an inflammatory response, may develop. In addition to the previously mentioned structures vulnerable to injury from abnormal pronation, the intrinsic foot muscles are now also at risk for injury as they contract vigorously to help stabilize the arch structure for propulsion. Excessive contractions may lead to fatigue and/or pain.

Hallux valgus deformity or bunions are likely to occur in the foot that is pronated during the propulsive phase. If the foot is pronated when the first MTP extends just before toe-off, a valgus force develops due to the abduction of the forefoot associated with abnormal pronation. This valgus force can be accentuated with improper shoe wear that has a narrow toe box, as in most women's and some men's dress shoes. As a result, the incidence of hallux valgus is much higher in women than men. Forefoot varus is the most common deformity that results in abnormal pronation during the propulsive phase.

A variety of other deformities and soft tissue abnormalities may contribute to abnormal pronation. For example, tightness of the gastrocnemius and soleus muscles may result in limited dorsiflexion of the ankle. If insufficient dorsiflexion is present during gait, the foot can obtain additional dorsiflexion at the oblique axis of the midtarsal joint. To obtain this additional dorsiflexion, the subtalar joint must be pronated to allow for midtarsal mobility. Factors that result in increased external rotation during gait can also result in increased subtalar joint pronation due to the body's center of gravity being further medial to the subtalar joint axis of motion as the body progresses over the foot during midstance. Common deformities in this category include external tibial torsion, femoral retroversion, and tightness of the hip external rotators.

Deformities at the hip and knee can influence foot mechanics as they affect the position of the foot relative to the ground at contact or by influencing the position of the foot with respect to the body's center of gravity at contact. For example, genu varum causes the medial aspect of the foot to rise further from the ground during contact. The foot must therefore pronate in order to be flat on the ground surface. Genu valgum, by contrast, results in abnormal pronation since it alters the body's center of gravity to a position in which it lies more medial to the subtalar joint axis, leading to increased torques and ultimately increased pronation.

BIOMECHANICAL TREATMENT FOR CONDITIONS ARISING FROM ABNORMAL PRONATION

Controlling abnormal pronation by voluntary muscle control has proven to be ineffective.[11] Therefore, the most common means of controlling abnormal pronation is via the use of biomechanical foot orthoses. These are prefabricated or custom-made shoe inserts that are constructed to conform to the foot when the subtalar joint is held in its neutral position. Control of abnormal pronation is obtained through midfoot support of the arch and in the forefoot and rearfoot by structures called *posts*. Posts are wedges added to the orthotic insert that function to "bring the ground up to the foot" and reduce the amount of compensation needed by the foot to get the plantar surface flat on the ground. For example, a foot that pronates late in the stance phase near toe-off can occur as a result of a forefoot varus deformity. With a forefoot varus deformity, we have noted that the medial aspect of the forefoot is elevated off the ground when the subtalar joint is in its neutral position (Figure 12-13). To "bring the ground up to the foot," a medial wedge can be added to the orthotic, thus reducing

or eliminating the distance that the medial forefoot must travel to achieve a position flat on the ground. This then indirectly reduces the amount by which the subtalar joint must pronate as a compensatory mechanism.

Abnormal Supination

Abnormal supination as a factor in overuse injuries occurs much less frequently than abnormal pronation. As mentioned earlier, the foot tends to compensate for deformities by pronating whenever possible, since supination requires a greater demand of energy. As a result, the abnormally supinated foot tends to be more rigid and is usually unable to pronate enough to compensate for deformities. During gait, the abnormally supinated foot will typically land with the calcaneus inverted and the subtalar joint in a supinated position. However, the subtalar joint stays supinated through the contact and midstance phases of gait. During propulsion, the foot may stay supinated or may demonstrate a late pronation at or near toe-off.[12] This late pronation occurs as a result of the foot being unstable laterally as the surface area of the foot in contact with the floor is reduced. An active pronation movement occurs to prevent the foot from rolling over laterally. The most common deformities associated with an abnormally supinated foot are forefoot valgus (an eversion deformity of the forefoot) (Figure 12-14), a rigid and plantarflexed first ray, and an uncompensated rearfoot varus. In an uncompensated rearfoot varus, the subtalar joint does not have sufficient motion to compensate for the deformity. This can be as a result of trauma, immobilization, or congenital factors.

The supinated foot tends to be rigid and does not pronate sufficiently, and as a result, its ability to attenuate shock is reduced. Therefore, many of the overuse injuries related to abnormal supination are due to the foot's limited ability to absorb shock or its acquired limited mobility. For example, calcaneal and tibial stress fractures may result from a rigid, supinated foot. Plantar fasciitis can also occur due to the significant tightness that exists in the plantar fascia following repeated stress to the calcaneal attachment, as seen with running activities. Finally, it is not uncommon for individuals with abnormally supinated feet to sustain repetitive inversion sprains to the ankle, especially during sporting events. The supinated foot has a tendency to be unstable laterally, and only a

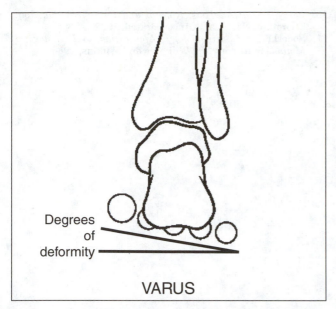

Figure 12-13. Schematic of forefoot varus deformity. Posting for this deformity consists of a medical wedge less than or equal to the amount of deformity.

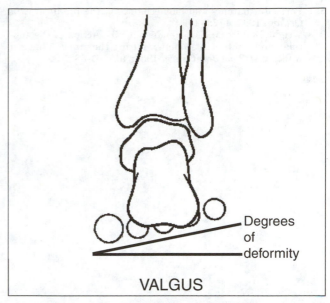

Figure 12-14. Schematic of forefoot valgus deformity. Posting for this deformity consists of a lateral wedge less than or equal to the amount of deformity.

slight change in terrain or sudden loss of balance is needed during single limb support for the ankle to turn over and sustain a lateral ankle sprain.

Lateral ankle sprains occur at a much higher frequency than medial ankle sprains. The lateral ligamentous complex is much more sparsely distributed and fails at much lower tensile loads than its medial counterpart. The medial ligaments support functions as a check reign to normal motion of the foot during gait. Therefore, it is designed to be much stronger, wider, and better developed to serve this function. On the other hand, the lateral ligamentous complex is a check reign to abnormal motion or stresses to the ankle and is not as strong or developed. Because of the morphological differences, forces or stresses that are easily absorbed by the medial ligamentous complex can often result in injury to the lateral ankle ligaments. Furthermore, the location of the lateral malleolus as compared to the medial malleolus is slightly more distal. This is observed clinically upon palpation and especially during passive movements of inversion and eversion. The more distal positioning of the lateral malleolus limits the amount of available normal eversion range of motion. This, in turn, also reduces the chances of medial ligamentous sprains as a result of excessive forces and range of motions.

BIOMECHANICAL TREATMENT FOR CONDITIONS ARISING FROM ABNORMAL SUPINATION

Due to the supinated foot s reduced ability to attenuate shock, foot orthoses used with the supinated foot should pay careful attention to this concern. Orthotic devices made from hard thermoplastics or graphite are contraindicated in the supinated foot unless a protective shock-absorbing material covers the device. Typically, an orthosis for a supinated foot includes a forefoot valgus post to reduce the need for the foot to compensate for this common deformity. The forefoot valgus post functions in the same way as the forefoot varus post, except it is a lateral wedge used to reduce abnormal supination. In individuals who sustain repeated inversion ankle sprains, a lateral flair of the heel portion of the orthotic device can be helpful in reducing the lateral instability that sometimes exists at heel strike.

References

1. Williams PL, Warwick R, Dyson M, Bannister LH. *Gray's Anatomy.* 37th ed. London: Churchill Livingstone; 1989.
2. Duckworth T. The hindfoot and its relation to rotational deformities of the foot. *Clin Orthop.* 1989; 177:39-48.
3. Norkin CN, Levangie PK. *Joint Structure and Function: A Comprehensive Analysis.* Philadelphia, Pa: FA Davis; 1983
4. Rocce C. The leg, ankle and foot. In: *The Musculoskeletal System in Health and Disease.* Hagerstown, Md: Harper and Row; 1980.
5. Hicks JH. The mechanics of the foot. *J Anat.* 1953; 87:345-357.
6. Root ML, Orien WP, Weed JH. *Clinical Biomechanics, Vol. II: Normal and Abnormal Function of the Foot.* Los Angeles, Calif: Clinical Biomechanics Corporation; 1977
7. Manter JI. Movements of the subtalar and transverse tarsal joints. *Anat Rec.* 1941; 80:397-409.

8. Perry J. Anatomy and biomechanics of the hindfoot. *Clin Orthop.* 1983; 177:9-15.

9. Wright DG, Desai SM, Henderson WH. Action of the subtalar and ankle joint complex during the stance phase of walking. *J Bone Joint Surg.* 1984; 46A: 61-382.

10. Perry J. *Gait Analysis: Normal and Patholical Function.* Thorofare, NJ: SLACK Incorporated; 1992.

11. Soderberg GL. *Kinesiology: Application to Pathological Motion.* Baltimore Md: Williams and Wilkins; 1986.

1. Identify the anatomical components of the ankle and foot complex on a lab partner.

2. Give an overview of how muscles of the ankle and foot are classified. Do these muscles have any commonalities with respect to neural innervation? Blood supply?

3. Describe each of the following components of the ankle and foot complex: upper functional unit, lower functional unit, forefoot, midfoot, hindfoot.

4. Demonstrate single plane motions that occur in the foot and identify the plane in which each motion occurs, as well as the axis of rotation for each.

5. Define triplane motion. Where can this be found?

6. What is the functional relationship of the subtalar joint and midtarsal joint?

7. Explain how the windlass effect and the metatarsal break work together to assist with normal foot function during gait.

8. Define the neutral position of the subtalar joint.

9. How does the subtalar joint function as a torque converter during gait?

10. List one example of abnormal pronation. Be sure to explain its cause and effect as it relates to gait.

11. Describe how orthotics are used as an intervention for abnormal pronation and supination of the subtalar joint. How does their use differ between abnormal pronation and supination?

STUDY QUESTIONS

12

CHAPTER 13

GAIT

Jeff G. Konin, MEd, ATC, MPT

OBJECTIVES

After completion of this chapter, the reader will be able to:

DIDACTIC

1. List and define the phases of gait.
2. Define the terms associated with gait.
3. Recognize the role various muscles play in normal gait.
4. Distinguish the roles that base of support and center of gravity play in gait.
5. Identify gait abnormalities and deviations.

PRACTICAL

1. Demonstrate the different phases of gait.
2. Measure cadence, step length, and stride length.
3. Identify compensatory mechanisms with abnormal and deviated gait.
4. Assess one's gait from anterior, posterior, and lateral views.

INTRODUCTION

The act of ambulating is often referred to as *gait*. This act incorporates a number of principles, terms, and concepts that are used to recognize what is said to be "normal gait." The process of understanding what normal gait is and how it occurs is essential to any clinician who chooses to assess abnormal gait. Like any other situation, being keenly aware of what is expected and normal makes for a smoother assessment of what may appear to be abnormal or deviated. With respect to gait, often times the abnormality or deviation that one is looking for may be complicated by more than one positional change, thus requiring a broad receptiveness on the clinician's behalf to allow for a more complex assessment.

Much can be said about the process of assessing gait. It requires the incorporation of a number of clinical skills. These skills include not only observational data, but also the ability of a clinician to listen to and understand a person's complaints, signs, and symptoms so that all of the pieces of the puzzle can be appropriately fitted together. It is the intent of this chapter to provide the practicing clinician with a broad overview of the phases of the gait cycle as well as some common gait deviations seen clinically. The reader is encouraged to utilize information learned throughout this text to assist in the understanding of gait. For a more comprehensive description of gait analysis, please refer to the list of suggested readings at the end of the chapter.

PHASES OF GAIT

The gait cycle is initially defined and broken down into two phases: *stance* and *swing*.[1-7] With respect to a single limb, the stance phase is when it remains on the ground for a period of time. When it remains in the air for a period of time, the limb is in the swing phase. The typical stance phase makes up approximately 60% of the gait cycle, with the swing phase consisting of the remaining 40%.

Using the traditional terminology of a gait cycle, each phase can be further broken down. The stance phase consists of components termed *heel strike, footflat, midstance, heel-off,* and *toe-off.* The swing phase consists of components termed *acceleration, midswing,* and *deceleration* (Table 13-1).

With heel strike, initial contact of the foot with the ground occurs. Typically, this involves the heel or calcaneus only. As the sole of the foot comes in

Table 13-1
Traditional Phases of Gait

Gait Cycle	
Stance	**Swing**
Heel strike	Acceleration
Footflat	Midswing
Midstance	Deceleration
Heel-off	
Toe-off	

greater contact with the ground surface, one enters a position of footflat. During footflat, a person's body begins to shift forward with momentum. The point at which the body weight moves centrally over the foot is referred to as midstance. As the body continues with its forward momentum, the heel eventually begins to lift off the ground in preparation for the next step, this is the component of heel-off. During heel-off, the majority of the body weight is now centered over the forefoot, especially the first ray. The final component of the stance phase occurs when one's toes leave the ground, or toe-off (Figure 13-1).

As mentioned, the swing phase involves the limb in space as opposed to being in contact with the ground. The first component of the swing phase is acceleration. During acceleration, the foot leaves the ground and moves anteriorly from a position of being slightly behind the body to being just under the body. When the limb is under the body, it is referred to as being in midswing. Finally, as it continues to move anteriorly and slows down in preparation for another heel strike, it is said to be in the deceleration component of the swing phase (see Figure 13-1).

During each component of the stance and swing phases, it is essential that the hip, knee, and ankle joints are appropriately positioned to allow for normal gait. Changes in these positions can result in abnormal gait or gait deviations that may or may not be able to be compensated for. Please refer to Table 13-2 for a comprehensive look at the normal joint positions during the phases of gait as they occur in the sagittal plane. It should also be noted that while a joint is in a certain position, it may in fact be moving in a very different direction. For example, from midswing to deceleration, the knee is in flexion during the entire movement. However, it is decreasing the angle of flexion as it decelerates, thus it is extending. This will be further discussed later in this chapter with the role of muscles.

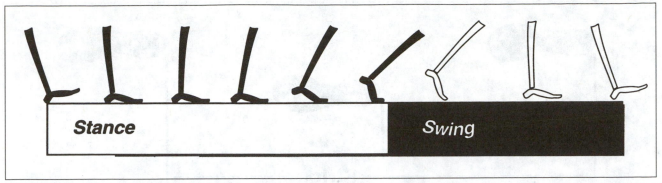

Figure 13-1. Divisions of the gait cycle. Limb segments show the onset of stance with initial contact, end of stance by roll-off of the toes, and end of swing by floor contact again (reprinted with permission from Perry J. *Gait Analysis: Normal and Pathological Function.* Thorofare, NJ: SLACK Incorporated; 1992).

Table 13-2
Joint Position During Gait: A Sagittal Plane Analysis

| | **Stance** | | | | **Swing** | |
	Heel strike to footflat	**Footflat to midstance**	**Midstance to heel-off**	**Heel-off to toe-off**	**Acceleration to midswing**	**Midswing to deceleration**
Ankle	Neutral to 15° PF	15° PF to 10° DF	15° DF	15° DF to 20° PF	PF to DF to neutral	Neutral
Knee	0° to 15° flexion	Extension to 10°	5° flexion	0° to 30° flexion	50° flexion	60° to 0° flexion
Hip	30° flexion	30° to 0° flexion	10° extension	Extension to neutral	30° flexion	30° flexion to neutral

PF = plantarflexion
DF = dorsiflexion

It is important to note that the traditional terminology of gait is not the only semantically accepted approach. Another approach, the Ranchos Los Amigos terminology, also exists. With the Ranchos approach, components of the stance phase include initial contact, loading response, midstance, terminal stance, and preswing. Components of the swing phase include initial swing, midswing, and terminal swing. Both methods can be appropriately used to identify one's gait cycle. However, we will refer to traditional terminology throughout this chapter.

ANALYSIS OF GAIT

There are many ways to look at how one's gait resembles a normally accepted gait, or whether it in fact deviates in any way. Beyond the positional movements previously described, there are also other variables that play significant roles during the gait cycle. These variables are related to time and distance.

Distance variables include stride length, step length, and base of support. Stride length is defined as the linear distance between two successive events that are accomplished by the same limb (Figure 13-2). Typically, heel strike is analyzed. One's stride length is equal to the heel strike of one limb to the very next heel strike of that same limb.[8] Average stride length has been found to be 1.46 meters (m) for males and 1.28 m for females[5] (Figure 13-3). Children will typically demonstrate a significant increase in stride length until they reach about the age of 11.[9] While a stride includes both a left and right step, it does not necessarily equate to the sum of each step since the distance of the left and right steps may differ. Other factors affecting stride length may include age, gender, height, and leg length.[10-17] Furthermore, as one's gait increases, so does the stride length.[18]

Step length is defined as the linear distance between heel strike of one foot to the very next heel strike of the opposite foot (see Figure 13-2). Therefore, during a gait cycle, there exists two step

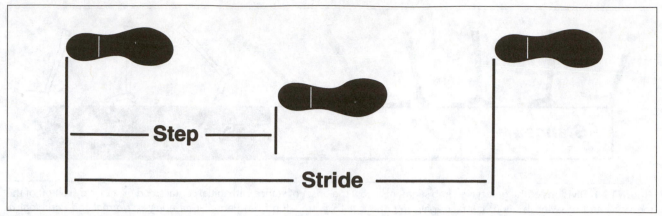

Figure 13-2. Step length and stride length (reprinted with permission from Perry J. *Gait Analysis: Normal and Pathological Function.* Thorofare, NJ: SLACK Incorporated; 1992).

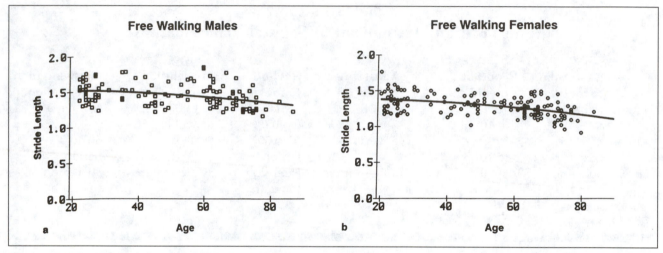

Figure 13-3. Normal stride length; a. males (N = 135); b. females (N = 158). Vertical scale = meters; horizontal scale = age (20 to 85 years) (reprinted with permission from Perry J. *Gait Analysis: Normal and Pathological Function.* Thorofare, NJ: SLACK Incorporated; 1992).

lengths: heel strike of the left to heel strike of the right, and heel strike of the right to heel strike of the left. These may not be equal, as mentioned previously, though the more equal they are, the more symmetrical one's gait will be with respect to linear distance.

One's base of support plays a large role in determining where one's center of gravity lies and subsequently his or her ability to balance during gait. The linear distance measured between the left and right foot is termed *the width of the base of support*. The average distance is considered to be between 1 to 5 inches and can vary with age, gender, and speed of ambulation. Increases in the width of the base of support will increase stability. In addition, when one's center of gravity is either lower to the ground and/or more centralized within one's base of support, a person's potential stability will increase with respect to balance.

During the gait cycle, the width of the base of support is influenced greatly by the speed of movement. During our discussion of the swing and stance phases, we have referred to each limb as either being in contact with the ground or in the air. When only one limb is in contact with the ground, the base of support is referred to as being in a *single limb support*. This is opposed to when both limbs are in contact with the ground, thus being in a *double limb support* position. During average speed of ambulation for walking, double limb support only occurs during approximately 10% of the gait cycle. Therefore, one can see that during single leg support, occurring 90% of the time during normal gait, the base of support is diminished greatly since there is only one point of contact with the ground. As one increases the speed of gait, the time spent in double limb support decreases further, requiring a greater effort to

Table 13-3
Muscle Activity During Gait

STANCE

	Heel strike	Footflat	Midstance	Heel-off	Toe-off
Hip					
Motion	Flexion 30°-25°	Flexion 30°-25°	Extension	Extension	Flexion
Muscle group	Gluteus maximus, hamstrings, addus magnus	Gluteus maximus, hamstrings	Quiet	Addus longus in late heel-off	Flexors
Contraction	Isometric	Isometric	Quiet	Eccentric	Concentric
Knee					
Motion	Flexion 5°	Flexion	Extension	Extension→flexion	Flexion
Muscle group	Quadriceps, hamstrings, popliteus	Quadriceps	Quadriceps→0°	Gastrocnemius popliteus	Gastro-nemius popliteus
Contraction	Eccentric (quadriceps) Concentric (hamstrings)	Eccentric	Concentric→0°	Eccentric→concentric	Concentric
Ankle					
Motion	Plantarflexion 0°	Plantarflexion	Dorsiflexion	Dorsiflexion→plantarflexion	Plantar-flexion
Muscle group	Dorsiflexors	Dorsiflexors	Plantarflexors	Plantarflexors	Plantar-flexors
Contraction	Eccentric	Eccentric	Eccentric	Eccentric→concentric	Concentric

SWING

	Acceleration	Midswing	Deceleration
Hip			
Motion	Flexion	Flexion	Flexion, extension at end
Muscle group	Flexors	Addus longus, gracilis	Extensors
Contraction	Concentric	Concentric	Eccentric
Knee			
Motion	Flexion	Extension	Extension→flexion
Muscle group	Hamstrings, sartorius, gracilis	Hamstrings	Hamstrings, quadriceps, popliteus
Contraction	Concentric	Eccentric	Eccentric→concentric
Ankle			
Motion	Dorsiflexion	Dorsiflexion	Dorsiflexion
Muscle group	Dorsiflexors	Dorsiflexors	Dorsiflexors
Contraction	Concentric	Concentric	Isometric/concentric

Adapted with permission from Perry J. Gait Analysis: Normal and Pathological Function. Thorofare, NJ: SLACK Incorporated; 1992.

remain in equilibrium.[19-29] During activities such as running, it is actually possible to find oneself in a position of no limb support, thus requiring tremendous ability to control the dynamic musculature during the deceleration component of swing as well as the heel strike component of stance.

The number of steps one takes per minute is called *cadence*. Average cadence is between 80 to 120 steps per minute. There is a wide variance in cadence since individuals have different styles in which they carry themselves. However, a significantly lower or higher cadence can indicate gait abnormalities. There is a direct relationship between cadence and limb support. As the cadence decreases, double limb support increases, providing greater stability. As cadence increases, as with running, double limb support decreases. Therefore, if one were ambulating with a significantly slow cadence, it might be suspected that he or she is purposefully attempting to increased double limb support for stability.

The time spent during each step is referred to as *step duration*. This too can indicate gait abnormalities or even injury. For example, any muscle weakness or injury to a limb might lead a person to spend less time on the effected limb, thus reducing step time. In turn, this may increase the step time on the contralateral limb.

ROLE OF MUSCLES

A number of muscles and muscle groups play a significant role in one's gait. Understanding the role of each muscle during each component of the different phases of gait helps to recognize the differences between normal and abnormal mechanics during gait (Figure 13-3).

Hip Joint Muscles

A number of muscle groups assist with movement and stability of the hip during the gait cycle. The hip extensors, especially the gluteus maximus, contract isometrically at heel strike in preparation to serve as a rigid limb.

As one moves through the stance phase, the activity of the hip extensors significantly decreases. The hip flexors also contract isometrically at heel strike and then begin to work eccentrically as one moves toward heel-off, thus slowing down the extension movement of the hip. During the beginning of the swing phase, the hip flexors work concentrically to accelerate the limb and then again eccentrically to decelerate the limb in preparation for heel contact.

Additionally at the hip, the medial and lateral stabilizers assist with maintaining balance during single leg support. This is highlighted with the gluteus medius acting in a reverse action role, helping to keep one's pelvis in a neutral position as a person moves through the stance phase. A weak gluteus medius will result in pelvic asymmetry in the frontal plane (Trendelenburg gait).

Knee Joint Muscles

The primary muscle groups acting at the knee are the quadriceps and hamstrings. The quadriceps muscles serve as knee extensors while the hamstrings serve as knee flexors. At heel strike, the quadriceps muscles contract isometrically as the knee prepares to withstand ground reaction forces. As the limb approaches midstance, these muscles work eccentrically while the goes into a flexion moment. From midstance to heel-off, little activity occurs. Then again at toe-off, the quadriceps begin to work eccentrically as the knee flexes in preparation for the swing phase.

Furthermore, as discussed in Chapter 12, the subtalar joint will take on a position of supination as the foot leaves the stance phase to allow for propulsion to occur. As the foot hits the ground and once again begins the stance phase, the subtalar joint moves into pronation and serves as a mobile adapter for the weightbearing forces.

During the swing phase, quadriceps muscle activity continues to be seen eccentrically during acceleration until the maximal flexion is achieved at the knee. At this point, the quadriceps briefly fire in a concentric mode to initiate the forward movement of the tibia. During deceleration, the hamstrings contract eccentrically to control the movement of the limb in the forward direction. Again, as the knee prepares for heel strike, the quadriceps contract isometrically to stabilize the knee joint.

Ankle Joint Muscles

As the foot approaches heel strike, the tibialis anterior, extensor digitorum longus, and extensor hallucis longus contract eccentrically as the foot moves into plantarflexion. Weakness of the above stated muscles would cause the ankle to plantarflex too much at heel strike, thus decreasing the ability of the foot to strike at the heel. This eccentric control remains to be seen in the ankle dorsiflexion muscles throughout footflat and midstance. Not until heel-off is a change seen. This change is quite rapid and involves the plantarflexor muscles such as the gastrocnemius, peroneus longus, flexor hallucis longus, and flexor digitorum longus to contract concentrically. This movement serves as the thrust for push-off prior to entering the swing phase.

The main action seen during the swing phase at the ankle is a contraction of the dorsiflexors strong enough to maintain the ankle in a neutral position that will allow for the foot to strike the heel in an optimal position. The plantarflexors do not contract to any significance during the swing phase.

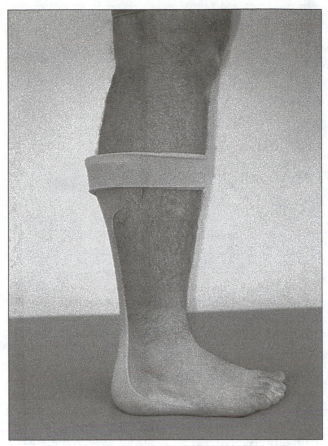

Figure 13-4. Ankle foot orthosis used to assist in dorsiflexion of the ankle.

GAIT DEVIATIONS, PATHOLOGY, AND PRACTICAL INTERVENTION

Foot Drop

Any disorder that leads to an inability to control adequate dorsiflexion of the ankle for clearance during the heel strike and swing components of ambulation is often referred to as a foot drop. Peroneal nerve palsy, weak dorsiflexors, decreased range of motion into the dorsiflexed position, or a plantarflexion contracture are conditions they may result in a foot drop. A person possessing any of the above mentioned conditions will typically enter the stance phase of gait with the initial contact occurring toward the forefoot, or he or she may make contact with the heel, which is followed by a rapid deceleration of the remainder of the foot.

The inability to control dorsiflexion also lends one to drag the foot on the ground during the swing phase. To compensate for this difficulty, a person may increase the amount of knee flexion or hip flexion to allow for adequate clearance of the foot. Essentially, the plantarflexed foot appears to make the involved limb longer than the noninvolved limb. One may also lean the trunk to the side to help carry the entire leg through the swing phase. In addition to strengthening the dorsiflexor muscles and stretching the heel cord, this type of condition may require an ankle foot orthosis to assist with the position of the ankle (Figure 13-4).

Weak Plantarflexors

A decrease in the amount of strength of the plantarflexor muscle group results in a decreased ability to push off the ground. This is seen during the toe-off component of the stance phase of gait and is referred to as a *calcaneal gait pattern.*[21] This is characterized by greater than normal ankle and knee flexion during stance and a shorter time spent in single leg support on the involved limb. Furthermore, the step length on the involved side may be shorter since the time spent in stance is reduced as a result of a diminished toe-off.

Inadequate Knee Flexion

Inadequate knee flexion may occur as a result of one having weak knee flexors, a knee extension contracture, or even an inability to control the relationship between the quadriceps and hamstring muscle groups during the gait cycle. Similar to a foot drop condition, the increased position of extension at the knee essentially lengthens the involved limb, making it more difficult to carry it through the swing phase. To compensate, a person may increase the amount of hip flexion or even circumduct the limb so that the foot does not drag through. Trunk extension is also a common movement that is increased with decreased knee flexion, in which one will lean backward by extending the trunk to allow for adequate clearance of the limb.

Knee Hyperextension

Hyperextension of the knee, or extension beyond 0° and the closed pack position, can occur from a number of conditions. Among these include weak quadriceps, weak hamstrings, joint instability, or joint flaccidity. Knee hyperextension is most influential during the heel strike and early stance components of the gait cycle. During this time, the knee does not serve as a rigid lever allowing for dispersion of ground reaction forces. Instead, the movement is directed slightly anterior and superior, thus increasing the potential for the knee to move into further hyperextension. This position is even more accentuated as one moves the upper body forward through the stance phase. Bracing the knee to help control stability is sometimes effective in controlling hyperextension of the knee during gait.

Weak Hip Flexors

While much of the movement for hip flexion occurs through passive momentum, it is still important to have strength in the hip flexor muscles both to maintain adequate hip flexion and for sagittal plane stability during the stance phase. Without adequate hip flexor strength, a muscle imbalance can lead to a difficulty in the eccentric movement while the involved limb returns to the ground. This will lead to a decreased swing time and possibly a more rapid heel strike. Strengthening of the hip flexor muscles and an assurance of proper flexibility in the antagonist muscle group can often times correct this problem.

Weak Knee Extensors

As previously mentioned, the quadriceps muscle group plays a key role in stability of the knee. Without the strong eccentric control of these muscles during heel strike, the knee would buckle since the center of gravity of the body falls behind the knee joint axis during this component of the stance phase. A person with normal hip extensor and plantarflexor strength can compensate for quadriceps weakness.[4] This is accomplished by forward bending of the trunk and rapid plantarflexion after the initial contact. This action creates an extension movement at the knee, thus moving the center of gravity more anteriorly and closer to a vertical plane with the knee axis.

Weak Gluteus Maximus

As a strong hip extensor, the gluteus maximus is responsible for controlling the forward movement of the hip during the early parts of the stance phase. Also, the gluteus maximus has been found to help control the femur by slowing down hip flexion during terminal swing. Both of these movements, occurring in the sagittal plane, are affected with a weak gluteus maximus muscle. During the stance phase, this can play a role in the stability one has

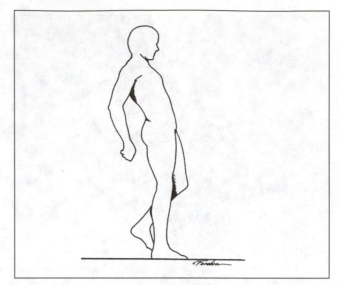

Figure 13-5. Backward lean of the trunk used to compensate for paralysis of the gluteus maximus muscle (reprinted with permission from Norkin CN, Levangie PK. *Joint Structure and Function: A Comprehensive Analysis.* Philadelphia, Pa: FA Davis; 1983).

during early stance. To compensate for this, one can maneuver the trunk in a posterior direction at heel strike in an attempt to re-align the center of gravity more posteriorly as well as preventing forward trunk movement. This is often referred to as a *backward lean* and is indicative of a gluteus maximus injury or weakness (Figure 13-5).

Weak Gluteus Medius

The gluteus medius muscle serves as a lateral stabilizer of the hip and pelvis, thus acting in the frontal plane. Weakness or injury to this muscle presents with a characteristic *Trendelenburg gait*. The main function of this muscle is to actually work in a reverse action, whereby it acts to keep the pelvis aligned in a transverse plane during unilateral stance. With a weak gluteus medius, one would exhibit a drop or lowering of the contralateral pelvis during single leg support. That is, if the left gluteus medius was weak, then during left limb single leg support, the right pelvis would appear to lower, beneath the transverse plane level of the left pelvis. This weakness not only produces a visible deviation, but it leaves one with a sense of instability in the frontal plane. To compensate for this feeling, a person will typically laterally bend the trunk toward the side of the weakness during the stance phase. This allows for a greater amount of stability since it returns one s center of gravity toward the central portion of the frontal plane.

Furthermore, it prevents any clearance difficulties one might experience during the swing phase of the uninvolved limb as a result of lowering of the entire limb toward the ground.

ENERGY COST OF AMBULATING WITH GAIT DEVIATIONS

There are some gait deviations that individuals may be able to overcome while attempting to ambulate, either by compensating with the use of certain muscles, re-aligning the center of gravity, or by using assistive devices. While these techniques may or may not present with a formally accepted approach to gait, they may be utilized by individuals as a means of being able to perform activities of daily living in the most practical way. One consideration that a clinician should keep in mind is the energy expenditure that one undertakes when modifying a gait pattern. For example, it may seem logical to set a high goal for a person who has suffered a spinal cord injury near the thoracolumbar region, such as to walk with the use of crutches and braces to help stabilize and support both lower limbs. Yet, the time required to prepare for the set-up and the amount of energy required to actually ambulate may be exhaustive to the individual. Depending on the person's physical condition, he or she may choose to bypass ambulation and instead maneuver in a wheelchair.

The same type of energy expenditures need to be considered when working with individuals who have musculoskeletal changes or any other pathological condition that may affect their gait pattern. Examples of these conditions may include those who have amputations, Parkinson's disease, hemiplegia, or surgical interventions, among others. Many studies have shown that the level of energy required increases, especially when one uses assistance of devices such as canes, crutches, or walkers.[22-35]

STEPS FOR ASSESSING GAIT DEVIATIONS

A complete assessment of gait involves many components that are essentially interdependent. Thus, understanding and recognizing only part of a problem or deviation may not provide the clinician with enough information to intervene with appropriate changes designed to improve one's overall function. Gait analysis can be performed in a clinical setting through mere observation, or it can be done with the utilization of computerized equipment that specifically measures movement patterns in a controlled laboratory. The ideal situation would be to have the benefit of both methods. However, most clinicians do not have access to the latter. Therefore, a number of steps have been identified to assist the practicing clinician with a sequential method of assessing gait. These steps have been designed to serve as a foundation, and further interpretation of findings may lead to additional inquiries deemed appropriate by the assessing clinician. These steps include:

1. Reviewing a person's current subjective complaints.
2. Reviewing any pertinent past medical history that may affect the condition or any part of the assessment.
3. Performing a preliminary observation of the individual's gait pattern to include weight-bearing status, use of assistive devices, and compensatory mechanisms.
4. Perform a physical assessment to include range of motion and strength, in particular.
5. Observing non-weightbearing and weight-bearing postures.
6. Carefully observing the individual's movement patterns during regularly paced walking. This should be done from an anterior, posterior, and lateral view.
7. Observing the patterns of wear on shoes, assistive devices, and anatomical contact surfaces.
8. Comparing subjective symptoms with physical signs and findings.
9. Making appropriate changes within reason.

Let us further explore these steps of gait assessment. Review of one's current subjective complaints is vital to understanding exactly why he or she has sought your assistance. It is the very reason why his or her life has been interfered with and has been faced with changes severe enough to disrupt activities of daily living. While an individual's comments are important and should always be respected, a careful review of past medical history should be performed. A clinician may find valuable data that describes possibilities of why certain pathology may exist. The piecing together of past medical history and current chief complaints should be done each and every time an individual is treated, as signs and symptoms may change, thus requiring a modification of treatment.

The preliminary observation is important, as it may be the only time in which an individual may not be as keenly aware that he or she is being looked at objectively. When a clinician asks a person to walk in front of him or her so that gait patterns can be observed, an individual may be so conscious of what is happening that he or she does not walk with a normal gait pattern. Whether or not this is intentional or accidental is not important. What is important is that the clinician is able to identify what is happening during the gait pattern under normal circumstances.

We have discussed in great detail how deficits in range of motion, or even excessive range of motion at a joint resulting in functional stability, may lead to pathology. Furthermore, strength deficits may also change the ability of one to ambulate under normal pain-free circumstances. Therefore, a full assessment of joint integrity, range of motion, and strength should be performed. When this is done prior to a clinician's critical observation of gait, it allows a clinician to formulate hypothesis as to why certain gait patterns may be affected. For example, if during a strength assessment a clinician makes a finding of weak dorsiflexors of a person's right ankle, the clinician may expect to see a foot drop gait during critical observation.

Throughout this text, many pathologies have been identified that can be directly related to improper biomechanics. Within the lower extremity, we have seen that deviations can occur in any plane and may, in fact, sometimes occur in more than one plane at a time. This is especially seen with triplanar motion of the subtalar joint. Since there are multiplanar possibilities of pathology, it is important that the clinician assess movement patterns from an anterior, posterior, and lateral view. These observations should pay careful attention to symmetry as well as findings that do not correlate to normal gait expectancies.

Observing the patterns of wear may indicate weightbearing patterns. For example, clinicians have historically analyzed the sole of the shoes for individuals who have complained of lower extremity pathology. One might recognize that the lateral rearfoot area of the sole may be wearing out at a faster rate than the medial side. While this finding may be significant, it does not necessarily indicate absolute and definitive deviations. For example, a wearing down of the lateral rearfoot area of a sole may indicate that an individual has a supinated foot. Or, it may simply indicate that the individual lands with the foot in a supinated position. This explains the importance of assessing joint position in both weightbearing and non-weightbearing situations. In the example previously described, the individual may actually have a pronated subtalar joint greater than normal, and in an attempt to compensate during ambulation and disperse forces, the individual excessively supinates.

Once all of the subjective and objective findings are gathered, information should be disseminated in a way that attempts to match the findings with the possible gait deviation. If a positive correlation is found, intervention can be performed with a sense of confidence. If findings appear somewhat gray, then further exploration of the situation may be indicated. All clinicians should remember that any change made, whether through the addition of an orthotic or change in weightbearing status, should be made in small increments. Changes made in small increments allow for an individual and the clinician to better assess the outcomes of the changes. Alterations that are made in increments too large may result in further exacerbation of the condition and may even create additional pathology. An example of a change made in too large an increment is the addition of an orthotic that has a rearfoot post that significantly changes the weightbearing status and foot positioning of an individual. A sudden change of the like may not be accommodating to the individual and thus become somewhat uncomfortable. This may be perceived as a failed approach to intervention, when in fact it may be the correct treatment intervention, only administered too rapidly.

References

1. Gould JA, Davies GJ. *Orthopaedic and Sports Physical Therapy.* St. Louis, Mo: CV Mosby Co; 1985.
2. Lehmkuhl LD, Smith LK. *Brunnstrom's Clinical Kinesiology.* 4th ed. Philadelphia, Pa: FA Davis; 1983.
3. Lippert L. *Clinical Kinesiology for Physical Therapist Assistants.* 2nd ed. Philadelphia, Pa: FA Davis; 1994.
4. Norkin C, Levangie P. *Joint Structure and Function.* Philadelphia, Pa: FA Davis; 1983.
5. Perry J. *Gait Analysis Normal and Pathological Function.* Thorofare, NJ: SLACK Incorporated; 1992.
6. Sarrafian SK. *Anatomy of the Foot and Ankle.* 2nd ed. Philadelphia, Pa: JB Lippincott; 1993.
7. Soderberg GL. *Kinesiology: Application to Pathological Motion.* Baltimore, Md: Williams & Wilkins; 1986.
8. Lamareaux LW. Kinematic measurements in the study of human walking. *Bull Pros Res.* Spring, 1971.
9. Beck RJ, Andriacchi TP, Kuo KN, Fermier RW, Galante JO. Changes in the gait patterns of growing children. *J Bone Joint Surg.* 1981; 63(A):1452-1456.
10. Das Rn, Ganguli S. Preliminary observations on parameters of human location. *Ergonomics.* 1965; 8:31-48.
11. Dean CA. An analysis of the energy expenditure in level and grade walking. *Ergonomics.* 1979; 22(11):1231-1242.

12. Grieve DW, Gear RJ. The relationship between length Of stride, step frequency, time of swing and speed of walking for children and adults. *Ergonomics.* 1966; 5(9):379-399.

13. Murray MP. Gait as a total pattern of movement. *American Journal of Physical Medicine.* 1967; 46:1.

14. Murray MP, Drought AB, Kory RC. Walking patterns of normal men. *J Bone Joint Surg.* 1964; 46A:335.

15. Shields SL. The effect of varying lengths of stride on performance during submaximal treadmill stress testing. *J Sports Med Phys Fitness.* 1982; 22:66-72.

16. Sutherland DH, Olshen R, Cooper L, Woo SLY. The development of mature gait. *J Bone Joint Surg.* 1980; 62A:336-353.

17. Winter DA, Quanbury AO, Hobson DA, et al. Kinematics of normal locomotion: a statistical study based on TV data. *J Biomech.* 1974; 7(6):479-486.

18. Larsson LE. The phases of the stride and their interaction in human gait. *Scand J Rehabil Med.* 1980; 12:107.

19. Inman VT. *The Joints of the Ankle.* Baltimore, Md: Williams & Wilkins; 1976.

20. Inman VT. *Human Walking.* Baltimore, Md: Williams & Wilkins; 1981.

21. Scranton PE, McMaster JH. Momentary distribution of forces under the foot. *J Biomech.* 1976; 9:45.

22. Annesley AL, Almada-Norfleet M, Arnall DA, Cornwall DW. Energy expenditure of ambulation using the Sure-Gait crutch and the standard axillary crutch. *Phys Ther.* 1990; 70:18-23.

23. Bard G. Energy expenditure of hemiplegic subjects during walking. *Arch Phys Med Rehabil.* 1963; 44:368.

24. Bard G, Ralston HJ. Measurement of energy expenditure during ambulation, with special reference to evaluation of assistive devices. *Arch Phys Med Rehabil.* 1959; 40:415.

25. Corcoran PJ. Effects of plastic and metal leg braces on speed and energy cost of hemoparetic ambulation. *Arch Phys Med Rehabil.* 1970; 51:69.

26. Corcoran PJ. Energy expenditure during ambulation. In: Downey JA, Darling RC, eds. *Physiologic Basis Of Rehabilitation Medicine.* Philadelphia, Pa: WB Saunders; 1971.

27. Corcoran PJ, Brengelmann GL. Oxygen uptake in normal and handicapped subjects in relation to speed of walking beside velocity-controlled cart. *Arch Phsy Med Rehabil.* 1970; 51:78.

28. Franks CA, Palisano RJ, Darbee JC. The effect of walking with an assistive device and using a wheelchair on school performance in students with myelomeningocele. *Phys Ther.* 1991; 71:570-577.

29. Gordon EE, Vanderwalde H. Energy requirements in paraplegic ambulation. *Arch Phys Med Rehabil.* 1956; 37:276.

30. Gussoni M, Margonato V, Ventira R, Veicsteinas A. Energy cost of walking with hip joint impairment. *Phys Ther.* 1990; 70:295-302.

31. Herbert LM, Engsberg JR, Tedford KG, Grimston SK. A comparison of oxygen consumption during walking between children with and without below-knee amputations. *Phys Ther.* 1994; 74:943-950.

32. Leihneis HR, Bergofsky E, Frisina W. Energy expenditure with advanced lower limb orthosis and with conventional braces. *Arch Phys Med Rehabil.* 1976; 57:20.

33. McBeath A, Bahrke M, Balke B. Efficiency of assisted ambulation determined by oxygen consumption measurement. *J Bone Joint Surg (Am).* 1974; 56:994.

34. Ralston HJ. Energy-speed relation and optimal speed during level walking. *Internationale Zeitschrift fur Angewandte Physiologie Einschliesslicn Arbeitsphysiologie.* 1958; 17:277.

35. Waters RL. The energy cost of walking of amputees: the influence of level of amputation. *J Bone Joint Surg (Am).* 1976; 58:42.

Suggested Reading

Inman VT. *Human Walking.* Baltimore, Md: Williams & Wilkins; 1981.

Perry J. *Gait Analysis: Normal and Pathological Function.* Thorofare, NJ: SLACK Incorporated; 1992.

Soderberg GL. *Kinesiology: Application to Pathological Motion.* Baltimore, Md: Williams & Wilkins; 1986.

1. Define the two phases of gait and the components of each.

2. How can a person's stride length and step length be affected by an injury?

3. How does the center of gravity change for a person who is involved in a sprinting activity?

4. Identify how different muscle groups play a role isometrically, concentrically, and eccentrically throughout the gait cycle.

5. How does the assessment of gait differ from the anterior, posterior, and lateral views? List an example of a gait deviation that can be seen from each view.

6. What type of intervention could be applied to help correct a gait deviation such as foot drop? Trendelenburg gait? Inadequate plantarflexion?

7. Design a program to assist a person who has inadequate knee flexion during the gait cycle. Which muscles would you strengthen? Which muscles would you stretch? Are there any other techniques you might implement that were not discussed in this chapter?

8. Would assistive devices be effective interventions for any of the gait abnormalities described in this chapter?

9. How might using an assistive device during ambulation increase the energy expenditure of an individual?

10. List the steps associated with gait assessment. What findings might you expect to recognize within each step?

MUSCLES

Legend

PA = proximal attachment
DA = distal attachment
A = action
N = nerve innervation

MUSCLES OF THE NECK AND SPINE

Platysma

PA: Upper pectoral and deltoid regions by bundles from superficial fascia
DA: Anterior fibers: depressor labii inferioris and depressor anguli oris muscles
Posterior fibers: angle of mandible
A: Depress lower jaw and lip
N: facial

Sternocleidomastoid

PA: Sternal head: anterior surface of manubrium

Clavicular head: superior surface, medial third of clavicle
DA: Lateral half of superior nuchal line of occipital bone
A: Unilateral: ipsilateral side bending and contralateral rotation
Bilateral: flexion of head
N: Spinal accessory, C2, C3

Longus Colli

PA: Vertebral bodies of C5 to T3
DA: Vertebral bodies of C2 to C4, transverse process of C5, C6
A: Unilateral: ipsilateral side bend and rotation
Bilateral: flexion of cervical vertebra
N: Ventral rami C2 to C8

Longus Capitis

PA: Anterior tubercles of transverse process of C3 to C6
DA: Inferior surface of basilar surface of occipital bone
A: Unilateral: ipsilateral side bend and rotation
    Bilateral: flexion of cervical vertebra
N: C1 to C4

Rectus Capitis Anterior

PA: Lateral mass of atlas
DA: Base of occipital bone anterior to foramen magnum
A: Flexion of head
N: C1, C2

Rectus Capitis Lateralis

PA: Superior surface of transverse process of atlas
DA: Inferior surface of jugular process of occipital bone
A: Ipsilateral side bend of head
N: C1, C2

Scalenus Anterior

PA: Anterior tubercles of transverse process of C3 to C6
DA: Scalene tubercle and ridge of superior surface of first rib
A: Unilateral: elevate first rib
    Bilateral: flexion of neck
N: Ventral rami C5 to C8

Scalenus Medius

PA: Posterior tubercles of transverse processes of C2 to C7
DA: Superior surface of first rib behind subclavian groove
A: Unilaterally: ipsilateral side bend and rotation of cervical vertebra
    Bilateral: flexion of neck
N: Ventral rami C3, C4

Scalenus Posterior

PA: Posterior tubercles of transverse process of C4 to C6
DA: Outer surface of second rib

A: Unilateral: ipsilateral flexion and rotation of cervical vertebra
    Bilateral: flexion of neck
N: Ventral rami C4 to C7

Rectus Capitis Posterior Major

PA: Spine of axis
DA: Lateral portion of inferior nuchal line
A: Extension, side bend, and rotation of head
N: Suboccipital

Rectus Capitis Posterior Minor

PA: Posterior tubercle of atlas
DA: Inferior nuchal line
A: Extension and side bend of head
N: Suboccipital

Obliquus Capitis Inferior

PA: Spine of axis
DA: Transverse process of atlas
A: Ipsilateral rotation of atlas
N: Ventral rami C1, C2

Obliquus Capitis Superior

PA: Transverse process of atlas
DA: Superior nuchal line
A: Extension and side bend of head
N: Suboccipital

Splenius Capitis

PA: Nuchal ligament, spinous process of C7 to T4
DA: Mastoid process
A: ipsilateral rotation of head, extend head
N: Dorsal rami C7 to T4

Splenius Cervicis

PA: Spinous process of T3 to T6
DA: Transverse process of C1 to C4
A: Ipsilateral side bend and rotation of head
N: Dorsal rami T3 to T6

Iliocostalis Lumborum

PA: Iliac crest
DA: Lower sixth to seventh ribs
A: Lumbar extension and side bend
N: Dorsal rami spinal nerves

Iliocostalis Thoracis

PA: Lower six ribs
DA: Angle of upper six ribs
A: Thoracic extension
N: Dorsal rami spinal nerves

Iliocostalis Cervicis

PA: Angle of third to sixth ribs
DA: Transverse process of C4 to C6
A: Cervical extension
N: Dorsal rami spinal nerves

Longissimus Thoracis

PA: Transverse processes of lumbar vertebrae
DA: Transverse processes of thoracic vertebrae, lower ninth to 10th ribs
A: Thoracic extension
N: Dorsal rami spinal nerves

Longissimus Cervicis

PA: Transverse processes of T1 to T5
DA: Transverse processes of C2 to C6
A: Cervical extension
N: Dorsal rami spinal nerves

Longissimus Capitis

PA: Transverse processes of T1 to T5
DA: Mastoid process
A: Contralateral rotation of head, extension of head
N: Dorsal rami spinal nerves

Spinalis Thoracis

PA: Spinous process of T11 to T12, L1 to L2
DA: Spinous process of T4 to T8
A: extension of vertebral column
N: Dorsal rami spinal nerves

Spinalis Cervicis

PA: Nuchal ligament, spinous process C7, T1 to T2
DA: Spinous process of C2 to C4
A: Extension of upper spine
N: Dorsal rami spinal nerves

Spinalis Capitis

PA: Transverse process of C4 to C6, T1 to T7
DA: Between superior and inferior nuchal line
A: Extension of upper spine
N: Dorsal Rami spinal nerves

Semispinalis Thoracis

PA: Transverse process of T7 to T12
DA: Spinous process of C6 to C7, T1 to T4
A: Extension of spine
N: Dorsal rami spinal nerves

Semispinalis Cervicis

PA: Facet of C4 to C7, Transverse process of T1 to T6
DA: Spinous process of C2 to C5
A: Extension and side bend of cervical spine
N: Dorsal rami spinal nerves

Semispinalis Capitis

PA: Facet of C4 to C7, transverse process of C7, T1 to T6
DA: Between superior and inferior nuchal line
A: Extension and ipsilateral rotation of head
N: Dorsal rami spinal nerves

Multifidus

PA: Transverse process of C4 to C7, T1 to T12, L1 to L5, and posterior sacrum
DA: Spinous process of vertebrae above origin
A: Aids with spinal extension, side bending, and rotation
N: Dorsal rami spinal nerves

Rotatores

PA: Transverse process of C2 to T12
DA: Lamina of vertebrae above origin
A: Unilateral: assists with vertebral rotation
    Bilateral: assists with vertebral extension
N: Dorsal rami spinal nerves

Interspinales

PA: Superior spinous process from C2 to lumbar region
DA: Inferior spinous process one level above
A: Assists with extension of spine
N: Dorsal rami spinal nerves

Intertransversii

PA: Transverse process cervical to lumbar region
DA: Transverse process one level above
A: Assist with side bend of vertebral column
N: Dorsal rami spinal nerves

MUSCLES OF THE ABDOMEN

External Oblique

PA: Iliac crest, abdominal aponeurosis
DA: Interdigitating slips from lower eight ribs and serratus anterior
A: Unilateral: ipsilateral side bend, contralateral rotation
     Bilateral: flexion of trunk
N: Ventral rami lower six thoracic, upper two lumbar

Internal Oblique

PA: Iliac crest, inguinal ligament, lumbar fascia
DA: Linea albea, last three ribs, costal cartilage
A: Unilateral: ipsilateral side bend and rotation
     Bilateral: flexion of trunk
N: Ventral rami lower six thoracic, upper two lumbar

Transversus Abdominis

PA: Iliac crest, inguinal ligament, costal cartilage
DA: Linea albea, abdominal aponeurosis
A: Compression of abdomen
N: Ventral rami lower six intercostals

Rectus Abdominis

PA: Pubic symphysis, crest of pubis
DA: Xiphoid process, costal cartilage of fifth through seventh ribs
A: Compress abdomen, flexion of pelvis and vertebral column
N: Ventral rami lower six intercostals

Quadratus Lumborum

PA: Posterior iliac crest
DA: Twelfth, transverse process of L1 to L4
A: Side bend of trunk, elevation of pelvis (reverse action)
N: Ventral rami L1 to L3

Diaphragm

PA: Xiphoid process, lower six costal cartilage, L1
DA: Central tendon of diaphragm
A: Expand thoracic cavity
N: Phrenic, C3 to C5

MUSCLES OF THE UPPER EXTREMITIES

Trapezius

PA: External occipital protuberance, superior nuchal line, nuchal ligament from spinous process of C7 to T12
DA: Distal third clavicle, spine of scapula, acromion
A: Elevation and upward rotation of scapula (upper fibers), adduction of scapula (middle fibers), and depression and upward rotation of scapula (lower fibers)
N: Spinal accessory, C3, C4

Latissimus Dorsi

PA: Spinous process of T6 to T12, iliac crest, lumbodorsal fascia
DA: Floor of bicipital groove of humerus
A: Adduction, extension, and internal rotation of humerus
N: Thoracodorsal C6, C7, C8

Rhomboideus Major

PA: Spinous process of T2 to T5
DA: Medial border of scapula between spine and inferior angle
A: Adduction and downward rotation of scapula
N: Dorsal scapular, C5

Rhomboideus Minor

PA: Nuchal ligament, spinous process of C7 to T1
DA: Root of scapular spine
A: Adduction and downward rotation of scapula
N: Dorsal scapular, C5

Levator Scapulae

PA: Transverse process of C1 to C4
DA: Vertebral border of scapula between superior angle and root of spine

A: Elevation and downward rotation of scapula
N: Dorsal scapular, C3, C4

Pectoralis Major

PA: Sternal half of clavicle, sternum to seventh rib, cartilages first through seventh of ribs
DA: Lateral lip of bicipital groove of humerus
A: Adduction, flexion, and internal rotation of humerus
N: Medial and lateral pectoral nerves, C5 to C8, T1

Pectoralis Minor

PA: Outer surface of upper margin of third through fifth ribs
DA: Coracoid process
A: Depression and downward rotation of scapula
N: Medial pectoral, C8, T1

Subclavius

PA: Upper border of first rib
DA: Inferior groove of clavicle
A: Depression of clavicle
N: Nerve to subclavius, C5

Serratus Anterior

PA: Outer surface of upper eighth through ninth ribs
DA: Costal surface of vertebral border of scapula
A: Abduction and upward rotation of scapula (protraction)
N: Long thoracic, C5 to C7

Deltoid

PA: Distal third of clavicle, superior surface of acromion, spine of scapula
DA: Deltoid tuberosity of humerus
A: Abduction of humerus (middle fibers), flexion, horizontal adduction, and internal rotation (anterior fibers), extension, horizontal abduction, and external rotation (posterior fibers)
N: Axillary, C5, C6

Subscapularis

PA: Subscapular fossa
DA: Lesser tuberosity of humerus
A: Internal rotation of humerus
N: Upper and lower subscapular, C5, C6

Supraspinatus

PA: Supraspinous fossa of scapula
DA: Superior facet of greater tuberosity of humerus
A: Assists deltoid with abduction of humerus, depression of humeral head, external rotation of humerus
N: Suprascapular, C5, C6

Infraspinatus

PA: Infraspinous fossa of scapula
DA: Middle facet of greater tuberosity of humerus
A: External rotation of humerus
N: Suprascapular, C5, C6

Teres Minor

PA: Dorsal surface of axillary border of scapula
DA: Inferior facet of greater tuberosity of humerus
A: External rotation of humerus
N: Axillary, C5, C6

Teres Major

PA: Dorsal surface of inferior angle of scapula
DA: Medial lip of bicipital groove of humerus
A: Extension, adduction, and internal rotation of humerus
N: Lower subscapular, C5, C6

Coracobrachialis

PA: Tip of coracoid process of scapula
DA: Medial border of humerus
A: Flexion and adduction of arm
N: Musculocutaneous, C5 to C7

Biceps Brachii

PA: Long head: supraglenoid tubercle of scapula
    Short head: coracoid process of scapula
DA: Radial tuberosity and bicipital aponeurosis
A: Flexion and supination of forearm, flexion of arm
N: Musculocutaneous, C5, C6

Brachialis

PA: Inferior two-thirds of the anterior surface of humerus
DA: Coronoid process and tuberosity of ulna
A: Flexion of forearm
N: Musculocutaneous, C5, C6

Triceps Brachii

PA: Long head: infraglenoid tubercle of scapula
Lateral head: posterior and lateral surface of humerus
Medial head: inferior and posterior surface of humerus
DA: Olecranon process of ulna
A: Extension of elbow
N: Radial, C6 to C8

Anconeus

PA: Lateral epicondyle of humerus
DA: Olecranon process
A: Extension of elbow
N: Radial, C6 to C8

Pronator Teres

PA: Humeral head: medial epicondylar ridge of humerus, common flexor tendon
Ulnar head: medial side of coronoid process of ulna
DA: Middle of lateral surface of radius
A: Pronation of forearm
N: Median, C6, C7

Flexor Carpi Radialis

PA: Common flexor tendon
DA: Base of second and third metacarpals
A: Flexion and radial deviation of wrist
N: Median, C6, C7

Palmaris Longus

PA: Common flexor tendon
DA: Transverse carpal ligament and palmar aponeurosis
A: Assists flexion of wrist
N: Median, C7, C8

Flexor Carpi Ulnaris

PA: Humeral head: common flexor tendon
Ulnar head: olecranon process and dorsal border of ulna
DA: Pisiform, hamate, base of fifth metacarpal
A: Flexion and ulnar deviation of wrist
N: Ulnar, C8, T1

Flexor Digitorum Superficialis

PA: Humeral head: common flexor tendon
Ulnar head: coronoid process of ulna
Radial head: oblique line of radius
DA: Medial and lateral sides of middle phalanges of second through fifth digits
A: Flexion of proximal interphalangeal (PIP) and metacarpophalangeal (MP) of second through fifth digits and flexion of wrist
N: Median, C7, C8, T1

Flexor Digitorum Profundus

PA: Medial and anterior surface of ulna, interosseous membrane
DA: Base of distal phalanges of second through fifth digits
A: Flexion of distal interphalangeal (DIP), PIP, and MP of second through fifth digits, and flexion of wrist
N: Median, C6, C7 to second and third digits
Ulnar, C8, T1 to fourth and fifth digits

Flexor Pollicis Longus

PA: Volar surface of radius, interosseous membrane, coronoid process
DA: Palmar base of distal phalanx of thumb
A: Flexion of interphalangeal (IP) and MP of thumb
N: Median, C8, T1

Pronator Quadratus

PA: Distal one-fourth of volar surface of ulna
DA: Distal one-fourth of lateral border volar surface of radius
A: Pronation of forearm
N: Median, C8, T1

Brachioradialis

PA: Proximal two-thirds of lateral supracondylar ridge of humerus
DA: Styloid process of radius
A: Flexion of elbow
N: Radial, C5, C6

Extensor Carpi Radialis Longus

PA: Distal one-third of lateral supracondylar ridge of humerus, common extensor tendon
DA: Dorsal surface of base of second metacarpal
A: Extension and radial deviation of wrist
N: Radial, C6, C7

Extensor Carpi Radialis Brevis

PA: Common extensor tendon, radial collateral ligament
DA: Dorsal surface of base of third metacarpal
A: Extension and radial deviation of wrist
N: Radial, C7, C8

Extensor Digitorum

PA: Common extensor tendon
DA: Bases of middle and distal phalanges of second through fifth digits
A: Extension of DIP, PIP, MP, and wrist
N: Radial, C7, C8

Extensor Digiti Minimi

PA: Common extensor tendon
DA: Dorsal surface of proximal phalange of fifth digit
A: Extension of MP of fifth digit
N: Radial, C7, C8

Extensor Carpi Ulnaris

PA: Common extensor tendon
DA: Medial side of base of fifth metacarpal
A: Extension and ulnar deviation of wrist
N: Radial, C7, C8

Supinator

PA: Lateral epicondyle of humerus, annular ligament, radial collateral ligament, and ulnar fossa
DA: Proximal one-third of lateral and anterior surface of radius
A: Supination of forearm
N: Radial, C5, C6

Abductor Pollicis Longus

PA: Posterior surface of ulna, interosseous membrane
DA: Radial side of base of first metacarpal
A: Abduction of CMC joint of thumb
N: Radial, C7, C8

Extensor Pollicis Brevis

PA: Posterior surface of radius, interosseous membrane
DA: Base of proximal phalange of thumb
A: Extension of MP joint of thumb
N: Radial, C7, C8

Extensor Pollicis Longus

PA: Middle one-third of posterior surface of ulna, interosseous membrane
DA: Base of distal phalange of thumb
A: Extension of distal phalange of thumb
N: Radial, C7, C8

Extensor Indicis

PA: Posterior surface of ulna, interosseous membrane
DA: Dorsal surface of proximal phalange of index finger
A: Extension of proximal phalange of index finger
N: Radial, C7, C8

Abductor Pollicis Brevis

PA: Transverse carpal ligament, scaphoid, trapezium
DA: Radial side of base of proximal phalange of thumb
A: Abduction of the thumb
N: Median, C8, T1

Opponens Pollicis

PA: Transverse carpal ligament, trapezium
DA: Radial side of first metacarpal
A: Rotation of CMC joint of first digit (opposition)
N: Median, C8, T1

Flexor Pollicis Brevis

PA: Transverse carpal ligament, trapezium
DA: Base of proximal phalange of thumb
A: Flexion of proximal phalange of thumb
N: Median, C8, T1
    Ulnar, C8

Adductor Pollicis

PA: Oblique head: trapezium, trapezoid, capitate, base of first metacarpal
    Transverse head: volar surface of third metacarpal
DA: Ulnar side of base of proximal phalange of thumb
A: Adduction of thumb
N: Ulnar, C8, T1

Palmaris Brevis

PA: Ulnar side of transverse carpal ligament
DA: Ulnar side of palmar aponeurosis
A: Deepens arch of hand (passive)
N: Ulnar, C8, T1

Abductor Digiti Minimi

PA: Pisiform, tendon of flexor carpi ulnaris
DA: Ulnar side of base of proximal phalange of fifth digit
A: Abduction of fifth digit
N: Ulnar, C8, T1

Flexor Digiti Minimi

PA: Transverse carpal ligament, hamate
DA: Ulnar side base of proximal phalange of fifth digit
A: Flexion of proximal phalange of fifth digit
N: Ulnar, C8, T1

Opponens Digiti Minimi

PA: Transverse carpal ligament, hamate
DA: Ulnar side of fifth metacarpal
A: Rotation of CMC of fifth digit (opposition)
N: Ulnar, C8, T1

Lumbricales

PA: Initiating from the tendons of the flexor digitorum profundus:
     #1: radial side to second digit
     #2: radial side to third digit
     #3: adjacent side to third and fourth digit
     #4: adjacent side to fourth and fifth digit
DA: Into extensor digitorum at the base of the distal phalanges of second through fifth digits
A: Flexion of second through fifth digits at MP joints, extension of second through fifth digits at DIP and PIP joints
N: Median, C8, T1, to second and third digits
     Ulnar, C8, T1, to fourth and fifth digits

Dorsal Interossei

PA: Initiating from adjacent sides of metacarpals
DA: #1: radial side of proximal phalange of second digit
     #2: radial side of proximal phalange of third digit

#3: ulnar side of proximal phalange of third digit
#4: ulnar side of proximal phalange of fourth digit
A: Abduction of second through fourth digits
N: Ulnar, C8, T1

Palmar Interossei

PA: #1: ulnar side of second metacarpal
     #2: radial side of fourth metacarpal
     #3: radial side of fifth metacarpal
DA: #1: ulnar side of proximal phalange of second digit
     #2: radial side of proximal phalange of fourth digit
     #3: radial side of proximal phalange of fifth digit
A: Adduction of second, fourth, and fifth digits
N: Ulnar T8, C1

MUSCLES OF THE LOWER EXTREMITIES

Psoas Major

PA: Transverse processes (anterior) and bodies of lumbar vertebrae
DA: Lesser trochanter of femur
A: Flexion of hip, flexion of trunk (reverse)
N: Branches of L2, L3

Iliacus

PA: Upper two-thirds of iliac fossa, iliac crest, base of sacrum
DA: At the lesser trochanter with the psoas major
A: Flexion of hip
N: Femoral L2, L3

Sartorius

PA: ASIS
DA: Superior, medial surface of tibia
A: Flexion, abduction, and external rotation of hip, aids with flexion and internal rotation of knee
N: Femoral L2, L3

Rectus Femoris

PA: AIIS
DA: Tibial tubercle via the patella ligament
A: Extension of knee, flexion of hip
N: Femoral L2 to L4

Vastus Lateralis

PA: Greater trochanter and lateral linea aspera of femur
DA: Tibial tubercle via the patella ligament
A: Extension of knee
N: Femoral L2 to L4

Vastus Medialis

PA: Medial linea aspera, tendon of adductor magnus
DA: Tibial tubercle via the patella ligament
A: Extension of knee
N: Femoral L2 to L4

Vastus Intermedius

PA: Upper two-thirds anterior and lateral femur
DA: Tibial tubercle via the patella ligament
A: Extension of knee
N: Femoral L2 to L4

Gracilis

PA: Inferior one-half pubic symphysis and superior one-half pubic arch
DA: Proximal medial surface of tibia
A: Flexion and internal rotation of hip, internal rotation of knee
N: Obturator L2, L3

Pectineus

PA: Pectineal line, surface of pubis between iliopectineal eminence and pubic tubercle
DA: Line extending from lesser tubercle to linea aspera
A: Adduction, flexion, and internal rotation of hip
N: Femoral L2, L3

Adductor Longus

PA: Anterior pubis between crest and symphysis
DA: Central portion of medial lip of linea aspera
A: Adduction and flexion of hip
N: Obturator L2 to L4

Adductor Brevis

PA: Lateral surface of inferior pubic rami
DA: Line extending from lesser trochanter to linea aspera
A: Adduction, flexion, and external rotation of hip
N: Obturator L2 to L4

Adductor Magnus

PA: Ischial tuberosity, rami of ischium and pubis
DA: Proximal to distal surface of linea aspera, adductor tubercle
A: Adduction of hip, flexion (upper portion), and extension (lower portion) of hip
N: Obturator L2, L3 (upper)
    Tibial L3, L4 (lower)

Gluteus Maximus

PA: Posterior gluteal line, sacrotuberous ligament, dorsal surface of sacrum and coccyx
DA: Gluteal tuberosity of femur, iliotibial band
A: Extension and external rotation of hip, extension of trunk (reverse)
N: Inferior gluteal L5, S1, S2

Gluteus Medius

PA: Outer surface of ilium from iliac crest to posterior gluteal line
DA: Lateral surface of greater trochanter
A: Abduction and internal rotation of hip
N: Superior gluteal L4, L5, S1

Gluteus Minimus

PA: Outer surface of ilium between anterior and inferior gluteal lines, margin of greater sciatic notch
DA: Anterior border of greater trochanter
A: Abduction and internal rotation of hip
N: Superior gluteal L4, L5, S1

Tensor Fascia Latae

PA: Anterior iliac crest, anterior ilium
DA: Middle one-third of iliotibial band
A: Assists with abduction, flexion, and internal rotation of hip
N: Superior gluteal L4, L5

Piriformis

PA: Anterior surface of sacrum, sacrotuberous ligament
DA: Upper border of greater trochanter of femur
A: External rotation of hip
N: Nerve to piriformis S1, S2

Obturator Internus

PA: Margin of obturator foramen
DA: Medial surface of greater trochanter
A: External rotation of hip
N: Nerve to obturator internus L5, S1, S2

Gemellus Superior

PA: Outer surface of ischial spine
DA: Medial surface of greater trochanter
A: External rotation of hip
N: Nerve to gemellus superior L5, S1, S2

Gemellus Inferior

PA: Superior portion of ischial tuberosity
DA: Medial surface of greater trochanter
A: External rotation of hip
N: Nerve to gemellus inferior L4, L5, S1

Quadratus Inferior

PA: Lateral margin of ischial tuberosity
DA: Quadrate tubercle and linea quadrata of femur
A: External rotation of hip
N: Nerve to quadratus femoris L4, L5, S1

Obturator Externus

PA: Outer margin of obturator foramen
DA: Trochanteric fossa of femur
A: External rotation of hip
N: Obturator L3, L4

Biceps Femoris

PA: Long head: ischial tuberosity, sacrotuberous ligament
     Short head: lateral lip of linea aspera, lateral supracondylar line of femur
DA: Head of fibula, lateral condyle of tibia
A: Extension of hip and flexion of knee
N: Long head: tibial L5, S1, S2
     Short head: common peroneal L5, S1, S2

Semitendinosus

PA: Ischial tuberosity
DA: Upper, medial surface of tibia
A: Extension of hip and flexion of knee
N: Tibial L5, S1, S2

Semimembranosus

PA: Ischial tuberosity
DA: Posterior and medial surface of medial tibial condyle
A: Extension of hip and flexion of knee
N: Tibial L5, S1, S2

Tibialis Anterior

PA: Lateral tibial condyle, upper two-thirds lateral surface of tibia, and interosseous membrane
DA: Medial and plantar surface of medial cuneiform and base of first metatarsal
A: Dorsiflexion and inversion of ankle
N: Deep peroneal L4, L5

Extensor Hallucis Longus

PA: Middle one-half of anterior surface of fibula
DA: Base of distal phalanx of great toe
A: Extension of great toe, assists with dorsiflexion of ankle
N: Deep peroneal L5, S1

Extensor Digitorum Longus

PA: Lateral tibial condyle, upper three-fourths of anterior surface of fibula and interosseous membrane
DA: Dorsal surface of middle and distal phalanges of second through fifth toes
A: Extension of second through fifth toes, assists with dorsiflexion of ankle
N: Deep peroneal L5, S1

Peroneus Tertius

PA: Anterior inferior surface of fibula
DA: Dorsal surface of base of fifth metatarsal
A: Dorsiflexion and eversion of ankle
N: Deep peroneal L5, S1

Gastrocnemius

PA: Medial head: posterior medial femoral condyle

Lateral head: posterior lateral femoral condyle
DA: Calcaneus vis calcaneal tendon
A: Plantarflexion of ankle, assists with flexion of knee
N: Tibial S1, S2

Soleus

PA: Posterior surface of head and upper one-third of fibula, middle one-third of medial border of tibia
DA: Calcaneus via calcaneal tendon
A: Plantarflexion of ankle
N: Tibial S1, S2

Plantaris

PA: Lateral supracondylar line of femur
DA: calcaneus via calcaneal tendon
A: Plantarflexion of ankle
N: Tibial S1, S2

Popliteus

PA: Posterior lateral femoral condyle, oblique popliteal ligament
DA: Posterior surface of tibia above soleal line
A: Flexion and internal rotation of knee
N: Tibial L4, L5, S1

Flexor Hallucis Longus

PA: Lower two-thirds of posterior surface of tibia, interosseus membrane
DA: Base of distal phalanx of great toe
A: Flexion of great toe, assists with plantarflexion of ankle
N: Tibial S2, S3

Flexor Digitorum Longus

PA: Posterior surface of body of tibia
DA: Plantar surface of base of distal phalanx of second through fifth toes
A: Flexion of PIP of second through fifth toes, assists with plantarflexion of ankle
N: Tibial S2, S3

Tibialis Posterior

PA: Lateral portion of posterior surface of tibia, upper two-thirds of medial surface of fibula, posterior surface interosseus membrane

DA: Navicular tuberosity, plantar surface of cuneiforms, cuboid, sustentaculum tali, and plantar surface of base of second through fourth metatarsals
A: Plantarflexion and inversion of ankle
N: Tibial L4, L5

Peroneus Longus

PA: Lateral tibial condyle, head and upper two-thirds of lateral surface of fibula
DA: Medial cuneiform, base of first metatarsal
A: Plantarflexion and eversion of ankle
N: Superficial peroneal L5, S1

Peroneus Brevis

PA: Inferior two-thirds of lateral surface of fibula
DA: Lateral side of base of fifth metatarsal
A: Plantarflexion and eversion of ankle
N: Superficial peroneal L5, S1

Extensor Digitorum Brevis

PA: Upper lateral surface of calcaneus
DA: First tendon joins with tendon of extensor hallucis longus, second through fourth tendons join with tendons of extensor digitorum longus
A: Extension of metatarsalphalangeal (MTP) of toes
N: Deep peroneal L4, L5, S1

Abductor Hallucis

PA: Medial process of calcaneus, plantar aponeurosis
DA Medial side of base of proximal phalanx of great toe
A: Abduction of great toe
N: Medial plantar S2, S3

Flexor Digitorum Brevis

PA: Medial process of calcaneus, plantar aponeurosis
DA: Middle phalanx of second through fifth toes
A: Flexion of MTP and PIP of toes
N: Medial plantar S2, S3

Abductor Digiti Minimi

PA: Lateral and medial processes of calcaneus
DA: Lateral side of base of proximal phalanx of fifth toe

A: Abduction of fifth toe
N: Lateral plantar S1, S2

Quadratus Plantae

PA: Medial head: medial surface of calcaneus
Lateral head: lateral border of plantar surface of calcaneus
DA: Joins tendons of flexor digitorum longus
A: Flexion of DIP of second through fifth toes
N: Lateral plantar S2, S3

Lumbricales

PA: First: medial side of flexor digitorum longus (FDL) tendon of second toe
Second: adjacent sides of FDL tendons of second and third toes
Third: adjacent sides of FDL tendons of third and fourth toes
Fourth: adjacent sides of FDL tendons of fourth and fifth toes
DA: With tendons of extensor digitorum longus into the medial side of the bases of the distal phalanges of second through fifth toes
A: Flexion of MTP and extension of IPs of second through fifth toes
N: Medial plantar S2, S3 (first), and lateral plantar S2, S3 (second through fourth)

Flexor Hallucis Brevis

PA: Medial portion of plantar surface of cuboid, adjacent portion of lateral cuneiform
DA: Medial and lateral side of proximal phalanx of great toe
A: Flexion of great toe
N: Medial plantar S1, S2

Adductor Hallucis

PA: Oblique head: bases of second, third, and fourth metatarsals

Transverse head: capsules of second, third, and fourth MTP ligaments
DA: Lateral side of base of proximal phalanx of great toe
A: Adduction and flexion of great toe
N: Lateral plantar S2, S3

Flexor Digiti Minimi

PA: Base of fifth metatarsal
DA: Lateral side of base of proximal phalanx of fifth toe
A: Flexion of fifth toe
N: Lateral plantar S2, S3

Dorsal Interossei

PA: Four arising with two heads from adjacent sides of metatarsals
DA: First: medial side of proximal phalanx of second toe
Second: lateral side of proximal phalanx of second toe
Third: lateral side of proximal phalanx of third toe
Fourth: lateral side of proximal phalanx of fourth toe
A: Abduction of second through fifth toes, flexion of MTPs and extension of IPs of toes
N: Lateral plantar S2, S3

Plantar Interossei

PA: Three arising from the bases and medial sides of the third, fourth, and fifth metatarsals
DA: Medial sides of the bases of the third, fourth, and fifth proximal phalanges
A: Adduction of third through fifth toes, flexion of MTPs and extension of IPs of toes
N: Lateral plantar S2, S3

TRIGONOMETRIC RELATIONSHIPS FOR RIGHT ANGLES

This information is used with permission from Rasch PJ. *Kinesiology and Applied Anatomy*. 7th ed. Philadelphia, Pa: Lea & Febiger; 1989.

For the convenience of students in dealing with problems of bone-muscle leverage, some of the elementary trigonometric relationships for right triangles are summarized below and on the next page.

A, B, and C are the points of a triangle; a and b are the sides opposite angles α and β, respectively; c is the hypotenuse, opposite angle γ, the right angle (Figure B-1).

1. The sum of the angles of any triangle is equal to 180°.

$$\alpha + \beta + \gamma = 180°$$

2. Two angles are called complementary when their sum is equal to 90°. In a right triangle, the two angles between the hypotenuse and the adjacent sides are complementary.

$$\alpha + \beta = 90°$$

3. The sum of the squares of the sides of a right triangle is equal to the square of the hypotenuse (Pythagorean theorem).

$$a^2 + b^2 = c^2 \qquad a^2 = c^2 - b^2$$

$$\sqrt{a^2 + b^2} = c \qquad a = \sqrt{c^2 - b^2}$$

4. The sine of an angle of a right triangle is equal to the side opposite divided by the hypotenuse and is equal to the cosine of the complementary angle.

$$\sin \alpha = \frac{a}{c} = \cos \beta = \cos (90° - \alpha)$$

5. The cosine of an angle of a right triangle is equal to the side adjacent divided by the hypotenuse and is equal to the sine of the complementary angle.

$$\cos \alpha = \frac{b}{c} = \sin \beta = \sin (90° - \alpha)$$

Below is a table of sines of the whole angles from 0° to 180°. The cosines of the angles may be found by taking the sine of the complementary angle, according to 5, above.

Degrees	Sines	Degrees	Sines	Degrees	Sines	Degrees	Sines
0 or 180	.00000	23 or 157	.39073	46 or 134	.71934	69 or 111	.93358
1 or 179	.01745	24 or 156	.40674	47 or 133	.73135	70 or 110	.93969
2 or 178	.03490	25 or 155	.42262	48 or 132	.74314	71 or 109	.94552
3 or 177	.05234	26 or 154	.43837	49 or 131	.75471	72 or 108	.95106
4 or 176	.06976	27 or 153	.45399	50 or 130	.76604	73 or 107	.95630
5 or 175	.08716	28 or 152	.46947	51 or 129	.77715	74 or 106	.96126
6 or 174	.10453	29 or 151	.48481	52 or 128	.78801	75 or 105	.96593
7 or 173	.12187	30 or 150	.50000	53 or 127	.79864	76 or 104	.97030
8 or 172	.13917	31 or 149	.51504	54 or 126	.80902	77 or 103	.97437
9 or 171	.15643	32 or 148	.52992	55 or 125	.81915	78 or 102	.97815
10 or 170	.17365	33 or 147	.54464	56 or 124	.82904	79 or 101	.98163
11 or 169	.19081	34 or 146	.55919	57 or 123	.83867	80 or 100	.98481
12 or 168	.20791	35 or 145	.57358	58 or 122	.84805	81 or 99	.98769
13 or 167	.22495	36 or 144	.58779	59 or 121	.85817	82 or 98	.99027
14 or 166	.24192	37 or 143	.60182	60 or 120	.86603	83 or 97	.99255
15 or 165	.25882	38 or 142	.61566	61 or 119	.87462	84 or 96	.99452
16 or 164	.27564	39 or 141	.62932	62 or 118	.88295	85 or 95	.99619
17 or 163	.29237	40 or 140	.64279	63 or 117	.89101	86 or 94	.99756
18 or 162	.30902	41 or 139	.65606	64 or 116	.89879	87 or 93	.99863
19 or 161	.32557	42 or 138	.66913	65 or 115	.90631	88 or 92	.99939
20 or 160	.34202	43 or 137	.68200	66 or 114	.91355	89 or 91	.99985
21 or 159	.35837	44 or 136	.69466	67 or 113	.92050	90	1.00000
22 or 158	.37461	45 or 135	.70711	68 or 112	.92718		

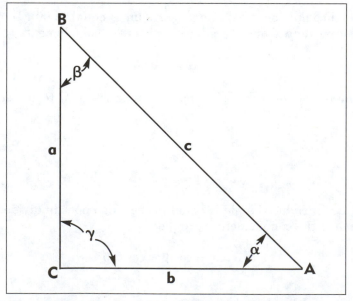

Figure B-1. Relationships of sides and angles in a right triangle.

*F*or your information

This book and many others on numerous different topics are available from SLACK Incorporated. For further information or a copy of our latest catalog, contact us at:

Professional Book Division
SLACK Incorporated
6900 Grove Road
Thorofare, NJ 08086 USA
Telephone: 1-609-848-1000
1-800-257-8290
Fax: 1-609-853-5991
E-mail: orders@slackinc.com
WWW: http://www.slackinc.com

We accept most major credit cards and checks or money orders in US dollars drawn on a US bank. Most orders are shipped within 72 hours.

Contact us for information on recent releases, forthcoming titles, and bestsellers. If you have a comment about this title or see a need for a new book, direct your correspondence to the Editorial Director at the above address.

*If you are an instructor, we can be reached at the address listed above or on the Internet at **educomps@slackinc.com** for specific needs.*

Thank you for your interest and we hope you found this work beneficial.